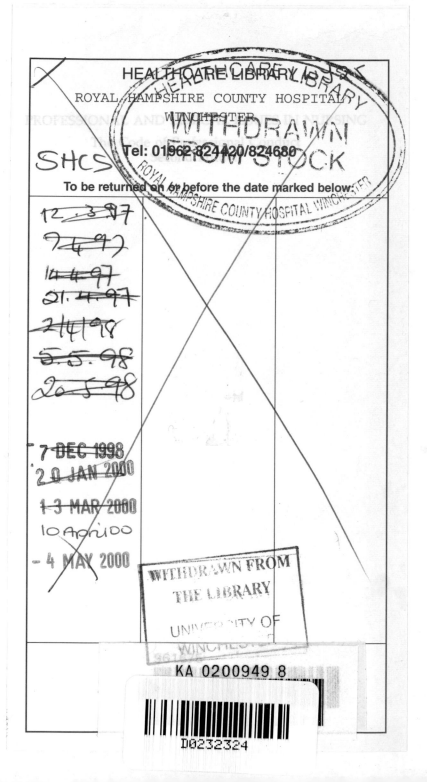

PROFESSIONAL AND ETHICAL ISSUES IN NURSING

The Code of Professional Conduct
Second Edition

# PROFESSIONAL AND ETHICAL ISSUES IN NURSING

## The Code of Professional Conduct

Second Edition

**Philip Burnard, PhD, MSc, RGN, RMN, DipN, CertEd, RNT**, Director of Postgraduate Nursing Studies, University of Wales College of Medicine, Cardiff

**Christine M. Chapman, CBE, BSc(Hons), MPhil, SRN, SCM, RNT, FRCN**, Emeritus Professor of Nursing Education, University of Wales College of Medicine, Cardiff

SCUTARI PRESS
London

Scutari Press is a division of Scutari Projects Ltd, the publishing company of the Royal College of Nursing.

First published 1993

**British Library Cataloguing in Publication Data**

Burnard, Philip
    Professional and Ethical Issues in
    Nursing:Code of Professional Conduct. –
    2Rev.ed
I. Title  II. Chapman, Christine M.
174.2

    ISBN 1–871364–96–5

Phototypeset by Intype, London
Printed by Bell and Bain Ltd., Glasgow

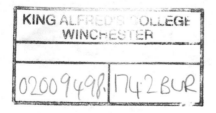

# Contents

# Acknowledgement

Thanks to Chapman and Hall, London, for permission to reproduce extracts from H. Wright and M. Giddey (1992) *Mental Health Nursing: From first principles to professional practice*.

# Preface

In 1988, we published the first edition of this short guide to professional and ethical issues in nursing. Since then, the UKCC has updated and revised the Code of Professional Conduct and we have updated the guide. Also, nursing has changed. We have seen the introduction of Project 2000, the development of primary nursing, the implementation of mentoring programmes and many other innovations and developments. In this edition, we have added sections on research, caring, the Data Protection Act, AIDS and mentoring and have generally revised the text.

As was the case with the previous edition, the guide is not meant to be a replacement for other books on ethics nor other books about nursing theory or nursing models. Instead, it is meant to supplement them by raising questions and initiating debate. Also, it is hoped that the book will be of value to midwives and health visitors. The Code, itself, is aimed at all three groups of people but the inclusion of all professional labels in the title of this book would make it clumsy! As appropriate, read 'midwife' or 'health visitor' for 'nurse' – although we are fully aware of and respect the differences between these professional groups. In the end, though, many professional and ethical issues apply across the board. This is not always the case but often it is.

Each chapter of this book examines one statement from the Code and explores the concepts and problems that relate to it. We do not suggest that what is discussed is exhaustive of what may be said on each issue, be we hope that the approach will act as a catalyst to debate and discussion.

The breadth of debate is also influenced by the perceptions of the authors which in many ways are very different: male and female, married and single, sociologist and psychologist, general nursing and psychiatry, Christian and searcher. However, what we have in common is that we are both nurses and both deeply concerned with the standards of care offered to the public, and to the development of the profession.

It is hoped that this new edition will be useful to a wide range of nurses, midwives and health visitors, Project 2000 students, nurse teachers and lecturers, managers and clinicians. As we have indicated, we do not claim to provide definitive answers – in the ethical field, they rarely exist – but we do hope to stimulate discussion.

*Philip Burnard*
*Christine Chapman*
1993

# INTRODUCTION

# Professional and Ethical Issues

This book is all about ethical and professional issues and this introduction explores the nature of ethics and professions as they relate to nursing. Both are addressed by the Code of Conduct. It is notable that the Code begins with the statement:

> Each registered nurse, midwife and health visitor shall act, at all times, in such a manner as to:
>> safeguard and promote the interests of individual patients and clients;
>>
>> serve the interests of society;
>>
>> justify public trust and confidence; and
>>
>> uphold and enhance the good standing and reputation of the professions. (UKCC, 1992)

These points summarise the issues that are at stake whenever ethical and professional issues are discussed.

## What is an ethical issue?

Living languages, like living people, constantly change; they develop, become more sophisticated, sometimes decay and may be abused. The word 'profession' is an example of the dynamic activity affecting words. At one time, to be a member of a profession meant one was either a member of the clergy, a physician or a lawyer; now it frequently means that the occupation so categorised is one requiring a degree of skill and/or specific knowledge. So we have professional footballers as well as professional engineers and architects.

In an early attempt to overcome the lack of a succinct definition of the word 'profession', Carr-Sanders and Wilson (1964) stated, 'the term profession . . . clearly stands for something. That something is a complex of characteristics'. Unfortunately, this statement

1

does not help a great deal as there is an absence of agreement as to what the characteristics are. Most lists of attributes, however, contain the following ideas:

A body of specific knowledge based on research.

For many years nurses were hesitant about claiming a specific body of knowledge. However, if, as Hockey (1974) asserts, nursing is a 'unique mix of knowledge and skills, many of which originated in other disciplines', then it may be said that nursing has a body of knowledge. Much of what nurses do has a theoretical basis which is not recognised or made explicit. For example, germ theory lies at the base of all aseptic nursing procedures: whether or not masks or gowns are worn; barrier nursing; lotions used to clean the skin or mouth and so on. The laws of thermodynamics and other related physical laws underlie procedures such as tem-perature-taking, tepid sponging and care of the hypothermic patient. Psychological theories have affected views on the visiting of children (and adults) in hospital, the relationship between infor-mation, anxiety and pain, talking to the dying patient and helping the bereaved relatives. Physiological theories should assist in the way in which medicines are given; assist the patient with elimin-ation and a great many more activities. Sociological theory contrib-utes to the understanding of the role of the patient and nurse; how organisations function; patterns of power and other social factors.

The qualifying statement 'based on research' is only gradually becoming true and, as the testing of knowledge increases, there is the exciting discovery that, in many cases, there is more than a 'mix' of knowledge as new knowledge is identified and syn-thesised.

> The amount and type of knowledge passed on to the new entrants to a profession and the specific skills required are directed by mem-bers of that profession, and the institutions involved in their edu-cation are validated by the profession.

This is certainly the case in nursing as the outline curriculum acceptable for registration is controlled by the United Kingdom Central Council and the four National Boards for Nursing, Mid-wifery and Health Visiting. In addition the approval of the edu-cational institutions and the qualifying examinations are the responsibility of the National Boards. Most professionals have their name entered onto a register of licensed practitioners. This register is important in that it conveys to the public not only that the individual has reached a satisfactory level of competence, but also that a certain standard of behaviour can be expected. This latter point is exemplified in the next characteristic.

The attitude of the professional towards the client is one of service on an individual basis, the clients' needs being placed before those of the professional.

In that the knowledge and skill possessed by the professional may be relatively difficult for the client to assess, there has to be an element of trust placed by the client in the professional which, in turn, the professional is prepared to accept. In order to reassure the client as to the standards of behaviour that can be expected, some professions have an ethical code which underlies their professional conduct. Deviation from this code may result in the professional's name being removed from the register of licensed practitioners.

Accountability for standards of practice is judged by fellow professionals and only they are able to make decisions as to whether the quality of service is appropriate.

However, Etzioni (1969) states: '. . . the ultimate justification of a professional act is that it is, to the best of the professional's knowledge the right act'. This demonstrates the high level of accountability that the professional must have for professional practice.

Public recognition is important to the professional and the phrase 'he's a real professional' is often used to indicate admiration of the skill demonstrated by the individual in a specific sphere of activity. The problem is that many people demonstrate a high level of skill in their job – consider the work of a diamond cutter or cabinet maker – yet these occupations are not normally considered professions. The level and type of knowledge underlying the skill and the relationship of the professional with the client are of a different order to that of the tradesman.

Professions tend to develop their own sub-culture.

Greenwood (1957) describes this as 'consciousness of kind' which binds members together. This may be demonstrated by the formation of a professional organisation which not only facilitates this coming together for mutual help and support but also, according to Greenwood, allows members to 'learn and evaluate innovations in theory. This provides a mutually stimulating milieu that is in marked contrast to the milieu of the non-professional'.

Such a list does not answer the question 'when is an occupation a profession?'. If an occupation is measured against such a list, how many positive 'ticks' are needed for the occupation to be called a profession? How many entitle it to be called a semi-profession? Where is the cut-off point?

As already stated, as far as the proverbial man in the street is concerned, it is the certainty of a particular type of behaviour that earns a person the title 'professional' rather than the possession by that occupational group of any number of characteristics.

It is for this reason that groups, recognised or not as professions, adopt codes of conduct by which members may be guided in their behaviour. Some codes are very old, an example being the Hippocratic Oath, variants of which are still taken by graduating medical practitioners, others such as the UKCC's Code of Professional Conduct are relatively new.

What is a code of conduct and what is its purpose and standing? What it is not, is law. This may come as a surprise to many people, especially as in many professions their code of conduct is used to judge professional behaviour and may be cited in disciplinary committees. A code of conduct is what it says it is, a code or guidance regarding appropriate conduct for a specific group of people carrying out specific actions. Many codes of conduct claim to be based on ethical principles (i.e. ICN Code for Nurses, 1973), others do not overtly make that claim but nevertheless have ethically based statements within their pages.

The definition of ethics is, like that of the word 'profession', fraught with difficulty. The *Concise Oxford Dictionary* states that it is the 'science of morals', which raises the question 'what is meant by morals?'. Tschudin (1986) claims that 'ethics is caring' and that 'to act ethically is to care . . . to care for ourselves and others'. This approach is certainly attractive to those who claim to be members of caring professions. However in a sense this approach is tautological and gives no real, practical guide to action. Indeed, the advocates of euthanasia often justify their claims to the right to end life on the basis that they 'care' and wish to relieve suffering, yet many would question whether such behaviour was ethical. In the place of the last word 'ethical' many people would substitute the word 'right' and it is the consideration of actions, beliefs and attitudes that makes up the study of moral philosophy. In an attempt to decide what is 'right', 'good' and 'just', Campbell (1979), in trying to separate out the difference between ethics and morals, acknowledged that the Greek and Latin from which the words derive mean roughly the same thing, 'that which is customary or generally accepted', but then went on to use the words 'morals' to describe the phenomena which are studied by 'ethics'.

The study of ethics may, therefore, be said to have two aspects. The first is related to how people 'should' behave and is based on the age-old debate engaged in by philosophers as to what is good, right and just. The second aspect, which can almost be considered to be the obverse side of the same coin, is related to what people actually do and the pressures – personal, cultural and organisational – which influence their action. The first consideration may lead to statements which ignore the consequences, the second sees the result of action as the most important factor. In making an ethical decision or in drawing up a code of conduct both aspects need to be considered.

Thiroux (1980) has established a set of principles of ethics which may be applied to any situation. They are:

1. The value of life.
2. Goodness or rightness.
3. Justice or fairness.
4. Truth telling or honesty.
5. Individual freedom.

It is important, according to Thiroux, to consider each of these principles when deciding on action. For example, if it is agreed that life is of supreme value, then when is it appropriate to stop striving to maintain it or when is death a realistic option? This is the first principle because without it the others are meaningless. However, Thiroux also states, 'human beings should revere life and accept death', which may help in making a decision to turn off a life support system. It may also help remind the nurse that quality of life has to be considered as well as quantity. Yet this fact produces another dilemma, the quality of life enjoyed by a severely handicapped person may, to the healthy young observer, appear to be very low indeed. To the person concerned life may still be precious and worth living.

The question as to the 'goodness' of an action has been debated since Aristotle, with a variety of measures being suggested by which an action may be judged. These range from original intention to the outcome of the activity.

Aristotle (see Chase, 1925) claimed that virtue lay in the appropriateness of the object or person for the task, so a 'good' knife is one that is sharp and cuts cleanly, because cutting is the function of a knife. It may also be aesthetically pleasing to look at or it may be ugly, valuable or of little intrinsic worth, but if it does its job, then it is 'good' and produces satisfaction or happiness. At first sight this is an attractive definition and may appear to solve the problem, but closer consideration will reveal some startling difficulties. What, for example, is the purpose of an individual, and can a person be described as 'good' because that purpose is met? The shorter Scottish Catechism states that 'the chief aim of man is to glorify God and to enjoy Him forever' and Benjamin Disraeli stated that 'man . . . is a being born to believe'. Whether or not you agree with these statements, or whether you prefer to substitute other functions as the purpose for the existence of human beings, it is easy to see that there may be individuals, perhaps physically or mentally handicapped, or aged and infirm, who are unable to perform the agreed function. Does this fact make them evil? Obviously not, so that while ability to function appropriately may be a useful way of assessing the value of a knife, it is no help in discussing the value of a man or woman.

Many people would say that everyone knows what is 'right' and 'good' by the way in which their conscience acts, making them feel that something should or should not be carried out. This is not a new idea. Bishop Butler writing in 1726 and cited in Roberts, 1970, developed an elaborate theory of conscience in which he claimed that having and obeying a conscience was essential to being classified as human. He explained this by comparing the human personality to a watch, whose separate parts are only of use when placed in relationship to each other. Conscience, he claimed, was an essential part of the mechanism of the human personality and without it the individual was incomplete. Further, he claimed that an individual was motivated by three factors. Firstly, by 'particular passions', that is, by basic drives like hunger, some emotional reactions such as fear and anger, and 'traits' like shyness or aggression. Secondly, by 'rational calculating principles', which calculate the individual's own long-term happiness, or what Butler called 'cool self-love', and the calculation of the happiness of others, which he described as 'the principle of benevolence'. Thirdly, 'conscience', which would hold the superior position and enable the individual to decide between the rightness of an action under the other motivating forces. For an individual to disobey his or her conscience, according to Butler, was to destroy the natural balance of his personality.

All this sounds fine, but of course people do not always obey their conscience. Another difficulty is that my conscience may say one thing and in an identical situation yours may dictate another. Indeed, it is this very conflict which causes so many problems in nursing/medical practice. One person fully believes that it is wrong to destroy life in any situation and therefore their conscience forbids them to assist with abortion; another believes, equally vehemently, that there are occasions when abortion is appropriate. Both must follow their own conscience and thus no consensus can be reached. Instead, to use Sartre's (1948) words, 'the individual is entirely alone and abandoned in his decision; he, and he alone, must take the responsibility'. Such a view cannot therefore be the basis of a code of practice to be followed by a group of people as each must make his own decision.

Another approach taken by a number of people when deciding on a course of action is to consider whether or not they would like it done to them. Charles Kingsley (1885) used this principle in his book *The Water Babies* when he created the character Mrs Do-as-you-would-be-done-by. Kant (1785) developed this point of view but also said that morality was doing one's duty for duty's sake. He described a series of actions as 'categorical imperatives'; that is, they must be followed. These are:

So act that the maxim of your action can become a universal law for all rational beings.

Act as if the maxim of your action were to become by your will a universal law of nature.

So act as to treat humanity, whether in your own person or in that of any other, in every case as an end, never as a mere means.

However, there are problems in applying this law of 'universality' when dealing with people who are themselves different and thus require different consideration. Does a commitment to preserve life mean that every patient who dies must be resuscitated because that is the universal law? Some would argue 'yes', while many would want to say 'it all depends'. Indeed, some would wish the patient to be given the opportunity to request that resuscitation should or should not be carried out, for, if this choice is denied, the patient may be used as a 'means' to enable the nursing or medical staff to comfort themselves with the thought that everything had been done for the patient. Yet Kant said that the person must be an 'end in himself'. Consider the arguments used to support the decision to spend money in one area of health care rather than another – remarks such as 'he is so young' or 'she is old and has had her life', heart transplants before treatment for arthritis, acute care before chronic, and so on. In all these statements 'ends' are implied regarding the worth of the individual in relation to their likely contribution to society: means, not ends in themselves.

The consideration of whether or not an action produces happiness may be more acceptable. Philosophers known as utilitarians, who may be represented by Jeremy Bentham and John Stuart Mill, assert that what is good is pleasure and happiness and what is bad is pain. A good action, therefore, is one that produces more pleasure than pain. However as any parent will know, a child's wish may often have to be denied, thus producing unhappiness, because granting the request may be dangerous for the child. Can such a denial be considered bad? A further problem is that happiness for one group may produce unhappiness for another. Who then is to be satisfied? The one with most power? So develops the tyranny of the majority.

From this discussion, it is obvious that it is difficult (perhaps impossible) to formulate one rule by which every situation may be judged, so that it can be said with certainty, 'this action is good, right and just'. One common thread running throughout the debate is the conviction that people cannot be treated as a collection of things such as knives and that each person has to be regarded individually. Indeed this is one of the first lessons learnt by the new entrant to nursing, and yet all patients must be treated alike.

Even this statement may be contentious: discussion as to whether an action is just or fair cannot stop at saying that all must be treated alike when it is quite clear that all are not the same to start with. Is discrimination, positive or negative, ever justified? We have already considered the problem in relation to expenditure on health care for specific groups. There is an apparent paradox in the statements 'all people must be treated alike' and yet 'each person has to be treated as an individual'. This paradox can be easily resolved: the nurse must not differentiate between patients on the grounds of colour, social class, education, attractiveness of personality and so on, only on the basis of the activity required to meet the patient's individual needs. However, this does not help the decision as to how to allocate scarce resources.

Schrock (1980) claims that nurses are often less than honest in their dealings with patients, yet honesty and truthfulness make up Thiroux's fourth principle. Most people in everyday life support varying degrees of honesty and truth telling. So much is this accepted that the telling of a 'white lie' carries little stigma on the basis that to do so may be kind. Can this ever really be justified? To what extent is the 'whole truth' necessary? Difficult questions, especially when caring for some patients, are nevertheless a principle of morality.

Another aspect of morality relates to the use of equipment and time. Both are easily misappropriated and thus the employer is defrauded. Yet how often is this considered stealing?

Finally, the principle of individual freedom. This, if present, will influence the way the first four principles are held and acted upon. What is more, it implies autonomy of action so that no one else can be held responsible for the actions of another. Nurses frequently question to what extent they have autonomy and, therefore, whether they can be held responsible for the care they give. Codes of conduct assume that the individual is accountable. To what extent are they correct?

What all this apparently leads to is a belief that a moral basis for action has to be rooted in the perception of the intrinsic worth of the individual and that person's right to self-determination. (Christians would back up this respect by explaining that man is created in the image of God.) The debate as to what constitutes a person has already been touched upon. Most agree that the definition includes the possession of an individual with humanoid characteristics, with a capacity, however small, to communicate and be communicated with (not necessarily by speech). 'Respect of person' in this context requires activity which is a combination of both rational and emotional elements used in a relationship of involvement with other individuals, so that their wishes, thoughts and aspirations are taken into account.

This approach, the respect of individuals, has some important implications. First, there is no final set of moral rules to guide action as modification may have to take place in the light of the individual; secondly, the individual is given greater value than society; thirdly, it demands an attempt to maintain an ongoing relationship with the individual, so that the person does not become an object to whom things are done. These factors are costly in time, resources and human endeavour and do not provide quick or easy answers.

It is in the light of this type of discussion that the United Kingdom Central Council for Nursing, Midwifery and Health Visiting (UKCC) issued, not a set of rules, but a Code of Professional Conduct as guidance for professional practitioners. The first Code specifically drawn up for those registered in the United Kingdom was published in 1983. This Code was circulated to the profession and comments requested. As a result of these comments a revised edition was issued in 1984 and another in June 1992.

It is interesting to consider why the UKCC has now produced a Code of Conduct when the International Council of Nurses produced their first code in 1953. The answer lies in the fact that while nurses in the UK previously used the ICN Code, the 1979

Nurses, Midwives and Health Visitors Act specified for the first time that the functions of the UKCC were to:

> . . . establish and improve standards of training and professional conduct . . . and that the powers of the Council shall include that of providing, in such a manner as it thinks fit, advice for nurses, midwives and health visitors on standards of professional conduct.

The provision of the Code has not been greeted with pleasure by all. Some of this displeasure has been due to misunderstanding of its function, fear that it might become a stick with which to beat the profession, and concern that it may be unrealistic in its demands. Certainly a great deal of concern expressed has been due to some of the guidance not being understood and the UKCC has attempted to increase understanding of some specific issues by the publication of explanatory leaflets.

Rumbold (1986) claims that professional codes serve three main functions:

1. To reassure the public.
2. To provide guidelines for the profession to regulate and discipline its members.
3. To provide a framework on which individual members can formulate decisions.

## The scope of professional conduct

Finally, the UKCC has made it clear how they plan to allow for the profession to expand. In 1992, they published a paper called *The Scope of Professional Practice* in which they outline how the profession might develop. Also, they laid down clear principles for adjusting the scope of practice which they maintain should govern any future expansion of the professional role of the nurse. These principles, drawn from the Code of Conduct itself, were:

The registered nurse, midwife or health visitor must:

1. Be satisfied that each aspect of practice is directed to meeting the needs and serving the interests of the patient or client.
2. Endeavour always to achieve, maintain and develop knowledge, skill and competence to respond to those needs and interests.
3. Honestly acknowledge any limits of personal knowledge and skill and take steps to remedy any relevant deficits in order effectively and appropriately to meet the needs of patients and clients.

4. Ensure that any enlargement or adjustment of the scope of personal professional practice must be achieved without compromising or fragmenting existing aspects of professional practice and care and that the requirements of the Council's Code of Professional Conduct are satisfied throughout the whole area of practice.
5. Recognise and honour the direct or indirect personal accountability borne for all aspects of professional practice.
6. In serving the interests of patients and clients and the wider interests of society, avoid any inappropriate delegation to others which compromises those interests.

It is with those principles in mind that we now turn to the Professional Code of Conduct itself.

## References

Roberts TA (ed) (1970) *Fifteen Sermons*. London: SPCK.
Campbell AV (1979) Plato. Apology 3A. In: *Moral Dilemmas in Medicine*. Edinburgh: Churchill Livingstone.
Carr-Saunders AM and Wilson PA (1964) *The Professions*. London: F. Cass.
Chapman CM (1976) The use of sociological theories and models in nursing. *Journal of Advanced Nursing*. **1**: 111–127.
Chase DP (trans 1925) *Aristotle, Nichomachean Ethics*. London: Dent.
Etzioni A (ed) (1969) *The Semi-Professions and Their Organization*. New York: Free Press.
Greenwood E (1957) Attributes of a profession. *Social Work*. **II**(3) 45–55. Washington: National Association of Social Workers.
Hockey L (1974) Forschung im Bereich der Pflege. Paper presented to Fortbildungskongress für psychiatrisches Krankenpflegepersonal und Sozialarbeiter, Heidelberg, Oct 1973. *Österreichische Krankenpflege Zeitschrift*. **27**(2) 41–48.
International Council of Nurses (1973) *Code for Nurses*. Geneva: ICN.
Kant I (1785) *Fundamental Principles of the Metaphysics of Morals*. (Trans. Abbott TK) New York: Library of Literal Arts.
Kingsley CC (1885) *The Water Babies*. London: Garland (1976 edn).
Mill JS (1869) *Utilitarianism*. London: Longman.
Nurses, Midwives and Health Visitors Act (1979). London: HMSO 50005.
Rumbold G (1986) *Ethics in Nursing Practice*. London: Baillière Tindall.
Sartre JP (1984) *Existentialism and Humanism*. London: Methuen.
Schrock R (1980) A question of honesty in nursing practice. *Journal of Advanced Nursing*. **5**(2) 135–148.
Thiroux JP (1980) *Ethics, Theory and Practice* (2nd edn). Cal: Glencoe Publishing Company Inc.
Tschudin V (1986) *Ethics in Nursing: The Caring Relationship*. London: Heinemann Nursing.

UKCC (1983, 1984 and 1992) *Code of Professional Conduct*. London: UKCC.
UKCC (1992) *The Scope of Professional Conduct*. London: UKCC.

# CHAPTER 1

# Promoting and Safeguarding the Interests of Patients

*Act always in such a manner as to promote and safeguard the well-being and interests of patients and clients.*

Considerable time and energy has been devoted to discussing the question 'what is nursing?'. It remains a favourite topic of debate at the beginning of Project 2000 courses as well as on higher nursing degree programmes. The answer to the question is complicated by the fact that nurses are not a homogeneous group of people, all engaged in virtually identical tasks. On the contrary nurses can be found in almost all walks of life: caring for infants and the aged; working in operating theatres and factories; in the midst of the battlefield; giving aid in famine stricken lands; providing highly technical care and teaching healthy living. So all-encompassing is the role of the nurse that it is tempting to answer the question 'what is nursing?' by saying that it is 'what nurses do'. However such an answer is to evade the purpose behind the question, which is to decide what, if anything, can be identified as the essential nature of the profession.

To answer this question it is important to consider not only the tasks performed by nurses but the motivation behind the tasks. One factor that is clear is that no matter where nurses work or what the nature of the task may be, nursing involves personal interaction between one individual – the nurse, and another individual – the patient or client. That is not to ignore the fact that sometimes the nurse is involved with a group of patients or that she may be part of a health care team; nevertheless at the point of contact it is individual with individual. Henderson (1966) defined nursing as:

. . . primarily assisting the individual (sick or well) in the performance

13

of those activities contributing to health, or its recovery (or to a peaceful death) that he would perform unaided if he had the necessary strength, will or knowledge. It is likewise the unique contribution of nursing to help the individual to be independent of such assistance as soon as possible.

Florence Nightingale (1859) was not happy with the word 'nursing'. She said that she used it for the want of another! However she described the work done by nurses as 'designed to keep people well, to help them to avoid disease, and to restore them to their highest level of health'.

What both these definitions have in common is that they focus on the individual patient or client, they stress the maintenance of health and the prevention of disease, and they emphasise the aim of patient independence.

The roles of nurse and patient are complementary. Without the presence of a patient there would be no need of a nurse (the word nurse in this context is used in its generic sense and therefore includes all branches of care provided by nurses).

## Becoming a patient

How does a person become a patient? Sociologists argue that this occurs in a variety of ways. Talcott Parsons (1966) suggests that a person has the right to be called 'sick' only if he seeks competent help, actively desires to get well and co-operates in the activity designed to assist in the return to health. In this case the individual is excused other roles. Certainly this is the way society works, in that it demands certification by a medical practitioner if the indisposition lasts more than a few days.

Robinson (1971), however, showed in his study of families in Swansea, that the presence of physical symptoms was not always sufficient to ensure that a person sought medical advice. Frequently, the difficulty of being excused social roles, the danger of losing a job if 'off sick', the problem of finding someone to care for children and other non-medical social factors, often meant that the person deferred or sacrificed the right to be classified as sick and failed to seek help.

It is always difficult to be certain why any person enters nursing, but when asked almost all say something to the effect that they want to help and care for people. Certainly the image that the public has of a nurse is of 'one who cares'. What is more they expect that this care will be of a personal nature, that is, the nurse will care for them not just as a 'patient' but as an individual. Jourard (1971) put it like this: 'one of the events which we believe inspires hope in a patient is the conviction that someone cares about him'. If this is true then the nature of the nurse/patient relationship is of prime importance. The problem is that most nurses find themselves working in an organisation which may have other aims than that of fostering effective interpersonal relationships, and this is true even of those who work outside traditional health care institutions. Melia (1981) found that most nurses were concerned with 'getting the work done' and it is often the fact that qualified nurses are rewarded for bureaucratic efficiency rather than for the quality of the care they provide. This is in stark contrast to the first guidance given in the Code which enjoins the nurse to 'act always in such a way as to promote and safeguard the well-being and interests of patients/clients'.

To be able to assess what are the interests of the patient or client the nurse has to have time to develop a personal relationship and to foster the feeling of empathy. The development of empathy requires the nurse to 'step into the shoes' of the patient in order to perceive the world through her eyes and to feel what she feels. Armed with this knowledge the nurse has then to return to the role of a nurse using the knowledge gained to enhance the care given. This does require that the nurse gets involved with the patient, an activity frequently frowned on in the past and still regarded with suspicion by many as being 'unprofessional'. What is unprofessional is an impersonal approach which results in all patients being treated as if they were identical, which is clearly not so.

To return to Jourard (1964), he observed that

> Much of contemporary interpersonal competence seems to entail success in getting patients to conform to the roles they are supposed to play in the social system of the hospital so that the system will work smoothly, work will get done faster and the patients will be less of a bother to care for.

What an indictment of a group of people who apparently entered the profession to care for others. The problem is that in some cases the nurse's desire to give physical care is such that the patient is not allowed to 'return to independence' even though that is an important aspect of care. Talcott Parsons (1966), in defining the role of the patient, said that not only must the person seek competent help and positively wish to recover, but also he must comply with the treatment offered. This may be appropriate but all care-givers need to remember that in the final analysis, the individual is responsible for his own life unless, as described by Henderson, he does not have the strength, knowledge or will.

## Advice

All health care professionals have problems accepting that the patient or client may not wish to accept the advice that they give. There is always the assumption that the doctor or nurse knows best, yet as the title of the famous play says, 'Whose life is it anyway?'.

Another important aspect of the role of the nurse in acting always in the best interest of the client is that of health educator. It is often felt that this is an aspect of care which is the sole responsibility of those specially trained for the task such as the health visitor or occupational health nurse. Nothing could be further from the truth. Nurses, by virtue of the respect with which they are held in society, and the fact that they are frequently in close contact with individuals and their families, are in a superb position not only to become involved in teaching healthy living but also, by their example, to demonstrate such living in practice. This is an awesome responsibility and should make any nurse who is obese or who smokes or who indulges in any other questionable life-style, stop and consider that by such actions the best interests of the client may not be served. It may be argued that just as clients have the right to self-determination in regard to their lives, so nurses have equal rights. In one sense this is true but, as already argued in the introduction, by belonging to a profession the nurse assumes certain responsibilities and in return is accorded special rights. Indeed rights and duties can be seen as the opposite sides of the same coin.

What is meant by the words 'right' and 'duty'? Benn and Peters (1959) argue that right and duty are different names for the same normative relationship (i.e. situation based on rules), varying according to the position from which the situation is regarded. In other words one person's rights become another person's duties. Rights also imply duties in another sense, in that the enjoyment by an individual of specific rights is usually conditional on the performance by that individual of specific duties.

## Rights and responsibilities

What then are the rights and responsibilities of nurses and patients when involved in patient care? The activity of nursing has undergone revision in the last 20 years: no longer is it seen as a collection of tasks performed on a passive patient but rather as a partnership between the nurse and the patient where both endeavour to achieve agreed health care goals. This implies an activity involving assessment, goal setting, planned intervention and evaluation of progress. All this is dependent on effective communication and interaction. Although, as already discussed, the nurse may have to act where the patient has not the strength, knowledge or will to act for himself.

The ICN Code for Nurses (ICN, 1973) denotes four main areas of responsibility for the nurse: to promote health, to prevent illness, to restore health and to alleviate suffering. Continuing the idea that one person's rights are another person's duties a picture emerges as shown in Table 1.1.

| Nurses' duties | Patients' rights |
| --- | --- |
| To promote health | |
| | Health |
| To prevent illness | or a |
| To restore health | peaceful |
| | death |
| To alleviate suffering | |

**Table 1.1** The four main areas of responsibility of the nurse

Stockwell (1972) also found that patients felt they had the right to receive:

1. Skilled care, 'a nurse you can depend on'.
2. Attention to 'trivial matters'.
3. More information.
4. More opportunity to voice worries and needs.

One of the responsibilities of the nurse is to act as the patient's advocate in situations where the patient is unable to act for herself. Advocacy is often a misunderstood concept. *The Concise Oxford Dictionary* defines it as '. . . one who pleads or speaks for another'. Patients frequently find it difficult to express fully their needs and fears. The nurse who has truly cultivated the skill of empathy and who is in frequent personal interaction with the patient may be able to interpret the patient's needs to others and to act as a go-between when other health care professionals appear, to the patient, to be unapproachable. This may also require the nurse to explain to the patient possible alternative lines of treatment and to ensure that the patient is fully aware of the implications before consent to treatment is given. This does not absolve other health care professionals from their responsibility to act in the best interest of the patient and most will do so, but it does place the nurse, who has this close, continuing relationship with the patient, in a special position of responsibility. Brown (1985) claims that 'advocacy is a means of transferring power back to the patient'.

| Nurse | | Patient | |
|---|---|---|---|
| Rights | Responsibilities | Rights | Responsibilities |
| *To have:* | *To give:* | *To receive:* | *To:* |
| Experience; | Skilled care; | Skilled care; | Co-operate; |
| Recognition; | Individual care; | Individual care; | Conform to |
| Reward; | Information; | Information; | routine; |
| Status; | Emotional support. | Empathy. | Be grateful. |
| Money; | | | |
| Gratitude. | | | |

**Table 1.2**   Rights and responsibility of the nurse and patient

## Earned rights

Curtin and Flaherty (1982) offer another slant on this debate. They suggest that nurses also have *earned rights* by virtue of the work they do, their experience in caring for others and as a result of their education and training. Among the earned rights they suggest nurses have are the following:

1. The right to practise nursing in accord with professionally defined standards.
2. The right to participate in and promote the growth and direction of the profession.
3. The right to be trusted by members of the public.
4. The right to intervene when necessary to protect patients, clients or the public.
5. The right to testify authoritatively to the community about the health care needs of people.
6. The right to be believed when speaking in their area of expertise.
7. The right to be respected by those inside and outside the

profession for their knowledge, abilities, experience and contributions.
8. The right to be trusted by colleagues.
9. The right to give to and receive from colleagues support, guidance and correction.
10. The right to be compensated fairly for services rendered.

In summary, Styles (1983) in her declaration of belief about the nature and purpose of nursing says: 'I believe in nursing as a humanistic field in which the fullness, self-respect, self-determination, and humanity of the nurse engage the fullness, self-respect, self-determination, and humanity of the client'. This is surely acting in the best interests of the client.

## Questions for reflection and discussion

1. To what degree do *you* think nursing ought to be a profession?
2. What are the implication of its *not* being one?
3. Has the fundamental nature of nursing changed over the last three decades?

### References

Benn SI and Peters RS (1959) *Social Principles and the Democratic State*. London: Allen and Unwin.
Brown M (1985) Matter of commitment. *Nursing Times* **81**(18) 26–27.
Curtin L and Flaherty MJ (1982) *Nursing Ethics: Theories and Pragmatics*. Englewood Cliffs, New Jersey: Prentice Hall.
Henderson V (1966) *Basic Principles of Nursing Care*. Geneva: International Council of Nurses.
ICN (1973) *Code for Nurses*. Geneva: International Council for Nurses.
Jourard SM (1964) *The Transparent Self*. New York: Van Nostrand.
Jourard SM (1971) *The Transparent Self*. 2nd edition. New York: Van Nostrand.
Melia KM (1981) *Student Nurses' Accounts of their Work and Training: a Qualitative Analysis*. Unpublished PhD Thesis, University of Edinburgh.
Nightingale, F (1859) *Notes on Nursing* (reprinted 1970) London: Dent.
Parsons T (1966) On becoming a patient. In: Folta JR and Deck ES (eds) *A Sociological Framework for Patient Care*. Chichester: John Wiley.
Robinson D (1971) *The Process of Becoming Ill*. London: Routledge and Kegan Paul.
Stockwell F (1972) *The Unpopular Patient*. London: Royal College of Nursing.
Styles M (1983) *Nursing: Towards a New Endowment*. St Louis: CV Mosby.

# CHAPTER 2

# Responsibility in Action

*Ensure that no action or omission on your part, or within your sphere of responsibility, is detrimental to the interests, condition or safety of patients and clients.*

The second article in the Code of Professional Conduct emphasises both the positive action and the negative omission side of the nurse's role and also points out that it may not be the nurse's direct activity that is under consideration but also the action of others within the sphere of influence.

> The ultimate justification of a professional act is that it is, to the best of the professional's knowledge, the right act. (Etzioni, 1969)

Implicit in this quotation is the idea that the professional person will take responsibility for the action because it is, in the specific circumstances, 'right'. Discussion has already taken place on the way in which the goodness or rightness of an action can be judged. The focus of this chapter shifts to the burden of responsibility or to adopt the term most frequently used these days, 'accountability'.

## Accountability and responsibility

The words 'accountability' and 'responsibility' are frequently used as if they were synonymous; however, there is a difference. While people may be held to be responsible for an action they may not always be asked to 'account' for it. The nurse however is not only responsible for the care given but should be able to explain why it was given in the way it was. It is necessary for the nurse not only to be concerned with the outcome of the action but also to understand its origin and the process of carrying it out. For example, a nurse may be responsible for getting a patient out of bed 12 hours after major surgery, however to be held accountable for this action implies that she has a reason for it, other than just that 'sister said so' and that the possible outcomes are understood. This means that the accountable nurse will understand the dangers of immobility and the incidence of deep vein thrombosis and also the possible unacceptable fall in blood pressure that may occur, thereby increasing the risk of shock. Understanding these possible results of not getting the patient out of bed she will make a decision as to the best course of action for that specific patient which may not be the same as the decision made for the patient in the next bed.

It is quite clear therefore that to be accountable requires knowledge so that the relative benefits or otherwise of alternative forms of action can be assessed. This means that while a student may be held responsible for care given to the patient, frequently it is not possible for the learner to be held accountable as she may not yet have the academic knowledge or the practical experience to assess the situation fully prior to carrying out the care. This has major implications in the use of the nursing process in that assessment of the individual patient is fundamental to all planning of nursing care. While it may be possible for a student to obtain and record information from the patient, the significance of the data, the identification of the nursing problems and the planning of care may have to be left to, or supervised by, the qualified nurse.

However it is not as simple as that. Knowledge should be research-based and up-to-date if it is to be 'the best', and this has implications for continuing education as a basis for accountability in practice. The requirement for the nurse to re-register every three years with evidence of the maintenance of professional knowledge is an attempt to ensure that all patients receive the highest level of care and that the qualified nurse can really be seen to be in a position to be accountable.

To be accountable also requires authority. It is of little value if the nurse knows what is the most appropriate method of care if some other person or circumstance prevents that care being given. Bureaucratic organisations often reject the idea of individual authority by insisting on 'chains of command', adherence to rules and policies, with no flexibility or discretion allowed to the individual practitioner. While it is easy to understand how managers, in assuming ultimate accountability for the total organisation feel in need of the protection of such rules, they are obviously less suitable in the health care setting where each client interaction is different from in a factory producing identical goods.

To summarise, to be accountable the nurse requires not only the appropriate up-to-date, research-based knowledge, but also the authority to act with a reasonable degree of autonomy. It is a waste of resources and a negation of expectations to prepare a nurse for three or more years to act in accordance with knowledge and to draw on experience gained in the clinical situation if individual judgment is then denied by either managerial style and/or tradition.

## Conflict

There are of course areas of potential conflict either between fellow nurses whose professional judgment may advocate alternative forms of action or between nurses and members of other professions. These situations are discussed later. In addition there may be conflict with the patient who has different expectations of what is appropriate care. This requires effective nurse–patient communication so that the patient understands the reason for the proposed action and the nurse understands the patient's point of view. If, however, having understood the action suggested and the likely outcomes of that and alternatives, or indeed no action, it is important to appreciate that in the end the patient has the final right of deciding on the care to be given or not given. In this case the nurse may have to surrender to the autonomy of the patient, who then assumes accountability for the decision. Nurses therefore are primarily accountable to their patients and then to their colleagues, the profession and the public.

When discussing accountability the emphasis is generally placed on 'doing'. However, it is equally important to appreciate that accountability also extends to 'not doing' and that omission of appropriate care is as serious as the performance of inappropriate care.

There is little doubt that for a nurse to fail to give a drug is a serious failure of care. Such an omission may prejudice the patient's chance of recovery, result in prolonged pain or lead to the development of organisms that are resistant to the drug. Equally negligent is the failure to record that the drug has been given as this may result in it being given again after too short a time interval.

Often health visitors feel that their actions are less open to abuse than those of nurses engaged in clinical practice. However, failure to carry out developmental tests on children, or failure to record the results of such tests, may prejudice the growth and development of a child.

At managerial level the failure to check that delegated responsibilities have been met may also be counted as negligence, as may failing to ensure that nurses have sufficient resources to carry out such tasks.

## Acts of omission

One specific act of omission that may occur is that caused by industrial action. Members of the Royal College of Nursing have rejected on many occasions the deletion of Rule 12 in the constitution which forbids such action, as they appreciate that it is not possible in the context of patient care. However in 1979 industrial action was taken by nurses belonging to other trade unions and as a result the then statutory body, the General Nursing Council for England and Wales, issued a statement as follows:

> The Council is of the opinion that if a nurse puts the health, safety or welfare of his or her patients at risk by taking strike or other industrial action he or she would have a case to answer on the score of professional misconduct, just as he or she would if the health, safety or welfare of patients were put at risk by any other action on his or her part.

Subsequent to this statement, in Northern Ireland, two charge nurses working in a psychiatric hospital were found guilty of misconduct by the GNC for 'absenting themselves from duty without good reason' during a strike called by the Confederation of Health Service Employees. During the case the chairman of the committee asked the members to consider the following questions:

1. Have the actions of the respondent damaged public confidence in the profession as a whole?
2. Have the actions resulted in actual or potential harm to any member of the vulnerable public?

On the evidence it was stated that one of the charge nurses was reluctant to strike but feared being labelled as a 'black leg'. While it is possible to understand that fear, especially when related to a comparatively closed community such as a psychiatric hospital, it is obvious that the chief concern of the nurse must be the safety of the patients in his care.

At the time the debate on the right to strike was hotly pursued.

Trade unions other than the RCN called the GNC's statement a threat, intimidation and blackmail. The then registrar of the GNC replied in an article published in *Nursing Mirror* in the following terms:

> The statement is not about taking industrial action, it is not about the nurses' right to strike, it is not about trade union activity, management/staff relationships, resource allocation or the many other issues which have arisen as a result of misinterpretation. It is about the health, safety and welfare of patients and the particular responsibility the qualified nurse holds in not placing the patient(s) at risk. (Storey, 1979)

She also referred readers to the ACAS Code of Practice under the heading 'Responsibilities – individual employee' which states:

> Some employees have special obligations arising from membership of a profession and are liable to incur penalties if they disregard them. These may include, for example, in regard to health safety and welfare, over and above those which are shared by the community as a whole.

A professional employee who belongs to a trade union should respect the obligations he has voluntarily taken on by joining the union. But he should not, when acting in his professional capacity, be called upon by his trade union to take action which would conflict with the standards of work or conduct laid down by his profession if that action would endanger:

1. Public health or safety.
2. The health of an individual needing medical care or other treatment.
3. The well-being of an individual needing care through the personal social services.

Such statements are clear and unambiguous, and while sympathy must be felt for nurses who are frustrated in their endeavours to obtain action from either their employers or the government it is obvious that consideration of the patient must come first.

It is important to consider when an action or omission may be considered to be a mistake based on professional misjudgment and when such action or omission is negligence. Brazier (1987) explains that:

> A nurse will be judged in accordance with the standard of skill and carefulness to be expected of a nurse in this position and speciality and with this seniority. A midwife must show a midwife's skill. It is not enough, for example, to display only the standard of an SRN who has done 13 weeks' obstetrics. A midwife holds herself out as a

specialist. . . . The more independent the nurse's function, the greater the risk of finding liability.

Although this last statement refers to midwives, nurses are also accountable and therefore may find themselves liable for negligence if they fail to follow instructions given to them by a physician or if they deviate from health authority policy. In some cases the negligence may be shared as in the cases where, while the nurse has not met the appropriate standard of care, management may also be at fault by not ensuring that resources and policies make that standard possible.

## Sphere of influence

The sphere of influence of the nurse is considerable. Not only does it encompass those with whom she has an explicit or implicit contract to provide care but also those who may ask for help and advice in an informal manner. Thus while the patient on the ward has to all intents and purposes entered into a relationship with the nurse which is similar to a contract, the neighbour who seeks advice over the garden fence also has the right to expect skilled professional information. True the nurse is not contracted to provide such information or help but once the task is accepted then there is a duty to ensure that it is completed in an appropriate manner. The nurse remains a nurse when practising nursing whether on or off duty, whether acting in a voluntary capacity or as a paid professional. Accountability for action is unescapable.

The accountability of those who teach nurses must, in the first instance, be to their students, although indirectly they are also accountable to patients and clients, since, if the material they teach is inaccurate or out of date, then the student may unwittingly give inappropriate or even dangerous care.

This prime accountability to students may bring the teacher into conflict with nurses in managerial positions who quite properly are accountable for providing an adequate supply of manpower to wards and other areas of care. The conflict arises in times of staff shortage when the manager may wish to utilise a student in their employee role to fill a need for a 'pair of hands' while the teacher may see that the student's educational needs require experience in a totally different clinical area.

Managers of care may find themselves in other situations when it may be difficult to decide with whom accountability lies. Bureaucratic institutions have many goals, and while it is probable that all who are employed in the Health Service have as a prime goal the welfare of the patients and clients using the service there are also the goals of efficiency and cost-effectiveness to be considered. In addition, as spenders of the money contributed in taxes by the whole community, the manager is in a sense accountable to the public at large. The balance that has to be maintained between these sometimes conflicting areas of responsibility is a difficult one. The danger is that the loudest voice will be the one that is heard and that in some cases the group that needs care the most will be the one most neglected. Nurses in managerial positions have therefore to be very clear as to their sphere of accountability, providing resources to enable others to fulfil their role of giving care while also being responsible in the expenditure of money.

Professional accountability is frequently a complex issue, however it is not one that can be laid aside. Once a member of the profession of nursing the nurse cannot escape this burden no matter what role is held.

## Primary nursing

A relatively recent approach towards accountability in nursing has been the development of *primary nursing*. This has become important as a method and philosophy of organising care. Manthie (1980) identifies the following principles of primary nursing:

1. The allocation and acceptance of responsibility for decision-making to one individual.
2. Individual assignment of daily care by case method.
3. Direct person-to-person communication.
4. One person operationally responsible for the quality of care administered to patients on a unit 24 hours a day, seven days a week.

The implications for nurses are clear: they not only have to think carefully about the way they plan and organise their nursing work but they also have to accept responsibility and accountability for that care on a long-term basis. Hegyvary (1982) summarises these and other points, thus:

1. Accountability: the primary nurse is answerable for the nursing care of a patient 24 hours a day throughout the hospital stay.
2. Autonomy: the primary nurse has, and acts on, the authority to make decisions about the nursing care of her patients in the mode of professional governance.

3. Co-ordination: nursing care is continuous around the clock with a smooth, uninterrupted flow from shift to shift and with direct communication from care giver to care giver.
4. Comprehensiveness: each care giver gives all required nursing care to a patient during a specific time period, e.g. a shift.

Strong claims have been made for the efficacy of primary nursing. Girvin (1991), for example, sees primary nursing as 'a revitaliser of the nursing profession'. Walsh (in Black 1992) argues that primary nursing will enable nurses to cope better with the larger numbers of patients being admitted and treated in hospitals and feels that it is more appropriate as a means of caring for short-stay patients. Research into primary nurses reports mixed findings and, as Black (1992) reports, it is too early to tell whether or not primary nursing will become the new 'norm' of how nursing work is organised. It is telling, perhaps, that Black identifies factors in the 'resistance to primary nursing' and that he identifies general 'resistance to change' as one of them. This suggests that primary nursing has already been established as a 'good thing' and that any resistance to it can be seen as a more general reluctance to change practice. Another approach might be to develop wide-ranging research projects to test the efficacy or otherwise of primary nursing before it is adopted as general strategy.

The reader who is interested in this innovative approach to the organisation of nursing care is recommended to read the key texts listed in the section on further reading.

## Questions for reflection and discussion

1. To what degree are *you* responsible for your actions?
2. What are your views on the appropriateness of primary nursing as an approach to organising nursing work?

### Further reading

Ersser S and Tutton E (1991) *Primary Nursing in Perspective*. London: Scutari Press.
Macdonald M (1988) Primary nursing: is it worth it? *Journal of Advanced Nursing* **13**(6) 797–806.
Macquire J (1989) An approach to evaluating the introduction of primary nursing in an acute medical unit for the elderly. 1: Principles and practice. *International Journal of Nursing Studies* **26**(3) 243–251.
Pearson A (1988) *Primary Nursing*. London: Croom Helm.

Vaughan B and Pillmoor M (1989) *Managing Nursing Work*. London: Scutari Press.
Wright S (1990) *My Patient, My Nurse*. London: Scutari Press.

## References

Black F (1992) *Primary Nursing: an introductory guide*. London: King's Fund Centre/The Foundation of Nursing Studies.
Brazier M (1987) *Medicine, Patients and the Law*. Harmondsworth: Penguin Books.
Etzioni A (1969) *The Semi-Professions and their Organisation*. New York: Free Press.
Girvin J (1991) Implementing primary nursing. *Nursing* 4(30) 522–533.
Hegyvary S (1982) *The Change to Primary Nursing*. St Louis: CV Mosby.
Manthie M (1980) *The Practice of Primary Nursing*. Boston: Blackwell.
Storey M (1979) Editorial *Nursing Mirror* 4th Oct. p. 4.

# CHAPTER 3

# Professional Knowledge and Competence

*Maintain and improve your professional knowledge and competence.*

At the moment, a considerable amount of basic nurse education is of the apprenticeship type. That is to say learner nurses work in the clinical situation and take time away from it for periods of study. Now at first sight this may seem to be a reasonable state of affairs: learner nurses gain practical experience alongside the theoretical inputs from the school of nursing. In practice, the situation is different. Schools of nursing can become detached from clinical practice, and staff working in the clinical situation (because of their own distance from training) come to view the school of nursing as idealistic or out of touch with reality. Nor is there evidence that the posts of clinical teacher or joint appointees (tutors with part responsibility as charge nurses) make any difference to this split between school and clinical area. Project 2000 (UKCC, 1986) is trying to change much of this but it is worth considering why such problems exist.

## Front-end model of education

One important reason for the theory–practice split may be the fact of nurse education's adherence to a 'front-end' model of education (Jarvis, 1983a). That is to say that the three years' training that leads to registration as a nurse currently comes in one lump at the beginning of the nurse's career. Figure 3.1 illustrates this diagrammatically.

Within this model, the nurse is deemed competent to enter the profession, fully, after the basic three years, and at present, is not

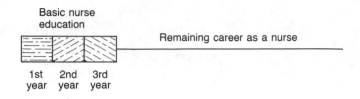

**Figure 3.1**   A front-end model of nurse education

required to undertake an educational course following that first three years, in order to continue to practise. It is notable that, at the time of writing, the UKCC is considering introducing compulsory 'refresher' courses for all trained nurses and has put forward proposals under a document called PREP. At present, many nurses do choose to pursue other educational courses and a wide range of such courses exists, ranging from two to three day workshops to Master of Nursing Programmes. The fact remains, however, that at present there is no obligation for the nurse to continue education after the first three years. (Most hospitals have a tutor with special responsibility for post-basic and continuing education but their task is a difficult one given the lack of obligation in the legal sense.)

There is, however, a moral obligation for the nurse to continue education. Alfred North Whitehead (1932), the philosopher of science, noted that 'knowledge keeps no better than fish!'. Knowledge soon becomes 'dead' knowledge: knowledge that is no longer relevant or accurate. The same can be said of skills. The skills learnt during basic nurse education are hardly likely to be sufficient throughout a nursing career. If the nurse is to remain a safe practitioner, knowledge and skills must be kept up to date.

While Project 2000 has led to a complete reshaping of the way in which nursing education is organised in Britain, the changes have also brought with them new initiatives for encouraging learning. Two examples of such changes can be mentioned before a more general discussion of keeping up to date is engaged in. A further discussion of the changes brought about by Project 2000 is also offered towards the end of this chapter.

First, *open learning* has come much to the fore. Various organisations have developed excellent material for helping people to learn at their own rate and often, through the post. Other initiatives in this field include open learning packages sponsored by nursing journals which have enabled many enrolled nurses to convert to registered nurse status. The Open University has also produced a number of well-thought-out open learning packages for nurses and these have enabled nurses to update their management, clinical and learning skills.

Second, *mentoring* has developed as a means of helping students to gain support in clinical settings and to encourage reflective practice in learning. Whilst the term 'mentor' has been the subject of considerable debate in the nursing literature (Atwood, 1979; Brown, 1984; Burnard, 1989, 1990a; Donovan, 1990), the notion of allocating students to a person who can act as guide and supervisor seems to be an important one and one included in the PREP recommendations.

Darling (1984) found in her research that there were three 'absolute requirements for a significant mentoring relationship'. These were: attraction, action and affect. In the first instance, attraction: it is deemed vital that both people respect and like each other. Arguably, as the relationship develops, a transference relationship will evolve (Burton, 1977). The term transference is usually reserved as a descriptor for the nature of the relationship which develops between a psychotherapist and her client. It signifies that the client comes to see the therapist as having personal characteristics (usually positive ones) that are reminiscent of one of the client's parents. All this normally takes place at a pre- or unconscious level so the client does not readily see that it is happening. The net result is usually that the client 'idealises' the therapist and becomes very dependent on her. One of the aims of therapy is often to help the client to try to resolve this transference relationship and thus live a less dependent and more interdependent life (Burnard, 1989). It seems likely that the relationship between student and mentor is also likely to invoke transference, particularly as the mentor is already cast in the role of 'expert' by the very nature of being a mentor at all. All this suggests that mentors should be chosen very carefully. Who should do this 'choosing' remains a question for debate.

The key issue seems to be learning to cope with perpetual change. Nursing, like many other professions and like the country itself, is in a constant state of change. It is vital, then, that all nurses learn to keep up to date. Indeed, the UKCC now sees such a process as mandatory. In future, nurses will have to give evidence that they have kept up to date in order to maintain their registration as nurses.

It is possible, too, that the 'attraction' could include emotional and sexual attraction. The ethical position, here, is clear – at least in theory. The relationship between mentor and student should remain 'platonic', given the tacit contract that exists between teachers, clinical staff and students. Life is rarely as simple as that, however, and the issue of how to cope with more involved relationships clearly needs addressing.

In terms of the 'action' role of the mentor, the student is likely to want to use the mentor as a role model. Again, by definition, the mentor is seen as an expert: someone who has achieved the various skills that are deemed necessary for effective practice and who is able to use and pass on those skills. In a sense, this aspect of mentoring may be equivalent to the 'sitting with Nellie' approach to training office staff in some organisations. 'Sitting with Nellie' refers to the idea of learning skills by sitting with and watching the person who has them. Clearly, though, it is to be hoped that this will not be the only way that skills are passed on. Traditionally, there has been an element of this approach in the past training approaches for students. Just being with a qualified person was sometimes seen as enough to encourage and enable students to develop skills. Whether or not this was ever the case is another debatable point! A certain skill in coaching seems to be a requirement of the skilled mentor. The ability to break down skills into component parts and teach them and then the ability to demonstrate their use with the appropriate, accompanying effect, seems to be another skill to aim for.

From the 'affective' point of view, the mentor needs to act in a supportive role. She should be able to encourage the student, enhance her self-confidence and teach her to be constructively critical of what she sees and does. Again, this aspect of the role is likely to re-open the debate about the likelihood of a transference relationship occurring. If it does and transference does occur, it is important that the mentor will be able to cope with it. She will also need to know how to close the relationship and be skilled in 'saying goodbye'. This is unlikely to be easy because of the possible 'counter-transference' that may occur: the mentor's complicated network of feelings for the student! At best, however, the relationship may come to mirror the best aspects of the truly therapeutic relationship that the student will develop with her patients. Hopefully, then, the mentor will be able to initiate and sustain the sort of exemplary relationship that will stand as a role model for future relationships. Again, a lot is being asked of the person who acts as mentor.

If such a relationship does develop and is sustained, it is likely to be very valuable for the student and, no doubt, for the mentor. If the heart of nursing is concerned with relationships, then a close relationship between one who 'knows' and one who is learning may be useful to both, and subsequently to the patients.

On the other hand, there are numerous problems. Because of the nature of the partnership, the student starts in a 'one-down' relationship with the mentor who is necessarily in a dominant position. It is not and cannot be a relationship of equals. Much of the recent writing on adult education has suggested that adult education should concern itself with negotiation, with shared learning and with meeting students' own perceived needs (Brookfield, 1987). The adult, so this argument goes, needs to use what he learns, as he learns it; he needs to be treated as an equal in a partnership that leads along a road of inquiry; he needs to have his self-concept protected as he goes. Whether such demands for equality and negotiation can exist within the constraints of the mentor–student relationship is not clear. It seems more likely that the mentor will be identified as a benign (or perhaps, not so benign!) father or mother substitute. Some may find such a portrayal overdramatic, but, as we have noted, the perfectly respectable notion of transference depends upon the 'unconscious designation' of the other person as a surrogate parent.

There is also the problem of the mentor's own development. There is nothing worse than the 'guru' who feels that she has gained enlightenment and all she needs to do is to sit back and pass on pearls of wisdom to others!

## Continuing education model

In order to consider the updating process, it may be useful to look at alternative models of education to the front-end model. Figure 3.2 illustrates the continuing education model.

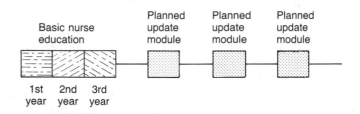

**Figure 3.2** A continuing education model of nurse education

In this model the three year basic education course is retained and planned modules are introduced at, say, yearly intervals. In this way, nurses continue the process of education throughout their careers. The objection may be made here that surely this model is the one offered by all hospitals that employ a post-basic or continuing education tutor. In fact, this is not the case. Post-basic education for nurses is rarely systematically organised in order that all nurses benefit from regular updating.

This model can be adopted by the individual nurse. Every nurse can, if she wishes, regularly review her own level of knowledge and skills and undertake to enrol on a post-basic course in order to make good any deficit. As we shall see, however, there are other ways of tackling the problem. Two obvious drawbacks to this approach may be noted. First, just because the individual nurse identifies particular learning needs does not mean that her desire to undertake a further course of study will necessarily be supported by her manager. Indeed, until further education for nurses becomes mandatory it seems likely that many nurses will not find support for further education activities. Second, the approach may be haphazard. It may be relatively easy to review knowledge and skills when a nurse feels highly motivated – it is not so easy after she has been qualified for a few years, and it possibly gets even more difficult as she gets older.

## Lifelong education

Figure 3.3 offers a second alternative: that of lifelong education. In this model, following a very short educational input to orientate the nurse within the profession, education itself is seen as a major part of the nurse's career, throughout that career. The lifelong education model acknowledges that all knowledge is temporary and subject to revision and must be modified in the light of research, personal experience and conceptual and theoretical changes. Skills are also viewed as evolving throughout the nurse's career. We do not learn a set of skills which somehow last throughout a working life but modify our skills, as we do our knowledge, through the light of professional and educational developments. Lifelong education is as much a philosophy or approach to education as it is a curriculum plan.

Lifelong education, as a philosophy for adoption by individual nurses or as a practical strategy for decisions about nurse education, may be adopted after further consideration about the nature of education itself. In order to make these further consider-

Educational activities

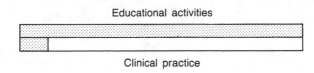

Clinical practice

**Figure 3.3** A lifelong education model of nurse education

ations, two ideal models of the curriculum are offered. An ideal model is one that sets out an example of the sorts of things that typify one approach. By curriculum is meant all those activities that go to make up the educational process: the setting of aims and objectives, the selection of materials for learning, methods of learning and evaluation methods. A typical curriculum model is illustrated in Figure 3.4.

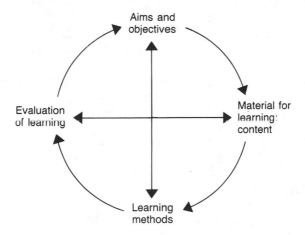

**Figure 3.4** A curriculum model

In this model, all aspects of the model relate to each other and the educational process is continuous. Education, then, is not something received once and for all but is a continuous, dynamic process of intellectual growth and development.

The two ideal models of the curriculum will now be described through reference to Table 3.1. The two curriculum models are

|  | Classical curriculum | Romantic curriculum |
|---|---|---|
| Basic focus of the educational process | Teacher-centred | Student-centred |
| Aim of the educational process | Teaching | Learning |
| Aims and objectives | Set by the teacher | Negotiated by teacher with learner |
| Contents of materials for learning | Decided by teacher | Evolved out of the relationship between teacher and learner |
| Learner methods | Predetermined by teacher | Decided upon by teacher and learner |
| Evaluation | Examinations set by teacher | Self- and peer-evaluation |
| Nature of knowledge concepts | Absolutist: 'facts exist' | Relative knowledge is dependent upon the one who knows |
| Similar education concepts | 'Banking' approach to education (Freire, 1980); pedagogy (Knowles, 1981) | 'Problem-posing approach' (Freire, 1980); andragogy (Knowles, 1981) |

**Table 3.1**   Two ideal models of the curriculum

known as the 'classical' and 'romantic' models. These terms have been used by a variety of writers, including the novelist Robert Pirsig (1976) and the educationalist Dennis Lawton (1973), who uses them to make comparisons between types of curricula in a similar way to the comparisons made here.

### Classical and romantic curricula

The two curriculum models offer very different views of the nature of education, and a closer examination of the differences between them may help to illustrate this. The classical model is teacher-centred and the aim of the model is teaching; that is to say that the teacher is perhaps a more important figure than the student. The teacher is seen as the 'one who knows' and the learner as the 'one who comes to learn'. The romantic model is student-centred and the main aim of the model is learning. Here, the teacher acts as a 'facilitator of learning' (Rogers, 1983). A facilitator is not a teacher but one who helps others to learn for themselves. A parallel may be drawn between the traditional nurse who 'cared' for the patient (who was a passive recipient of that care) and the modern nurse who is concerned with enabling the patient to care for himself. So it is in education. In the classical model, the teacher teaches: in the romantic model, the teacher facilitates learning.

Many things follow from this basic difference. In the classical model, aims and objectives are pre-set by the teacher. Lessons are pre-planned independently of the students and the teacher draws up the overall timetable. In the romantic model, aims and objectives are negotiated with the students: student needs and wants are identified, and lessons and the timetable are built around them. So it is with learning methods. In the classical model teaching methods are determined by the teacher. In the romantic model they are chosen through collaboration with the student in order that the student's needs are most suitably met. Evaluation in the classical model is by the use of tests and examinations, pre-set by the teacher. The teacher, having taught, wishes to find out if the learner has learned! In the romantic model both teacher and students engage in self- and peer-evaluation methods (Kilty, 1981; Burnard, 1987) whereby each learner (and teacher) assesses her own performance through a 'block' or term and then receives feedback on her performance from colleagues.

In this way it will be seen that the classical model involves 'teaching from above' whilst the romantic model involves the 'education of equals' (Jarvis, 1983b). In the romantic model both teacher and students are 'fellow travellers', for, as we see from the chart, the view of knowledge is one of relativism. Knowledge is something that grows out of the information and experience that is personal to each individual. Because each person views the world differently from other people, so individual 'knowledge' of the world will be different. In the classical model, knowledge is not relative: there are 'facts' out there in the world that are discernible. It is the teacher's task to pass on those facts. Thus, in the classical model, knowledge is 'impartial' and is unchanged by the one who knows it (Peters, 1969).

A distinction similar to the classical–romantic comparison is made by Paulo Freire (1970) when he describes the 'banking' concept of education versus the 'problem-posing' concept. The banking concept involves the teacher filling the students with information which is then 'cashed out' during examinations. In this model, 'more' knowledge is virtually equivalent to 'better educated'. Alternatively, the problem-posing approach is a means of education through dialogue. Teacher and student meet and exchange ideas through a heated, critical debate. Neither teacher nor student has the 'right' answer: there is room for a variety of possibilities.

Malcolm Knowles, the American educator, has used the term andragogy to describe negotiated adult-education as opposed to pedagogy or prescribed child-education (Knowles, 1981). Knowles argues that negotiated learning is that most appropriate for adults because of (a) the wealth of personal experience that they bring to the learning situation, (b) the fragile nature of their self-concept and (c) their need to use what they learn in a practical sense. As nurses begin their training at 18 years of age, it is clear that all nurses begin as adults and therefore Knowles' concept of andragogy may have much value in nurse education (Burnard, 1985). It is certainly possible to argue that traditional nurse education has tended to be of the classical, banking type and since modern nursing's aim is to produce the more autonomous patient, it would seem reasonable to argue for an educational system that gave nurse learners more control over their educational process. It seems difficult to see how autonomy in nursing can be encouraged unless there is also a degree of learner autonomy in nurse education.

On the other hand, it needs to be said that Knowles' principles of andragogy are not based on *empirical* work, but more on Knowles' own experience as an educator and on his reading of the literature. Many of his ideas can be traced back to the liberal educational philosophies of the American philosopher of science, John Dewey. Whilst there is much value in debate of this kind, it is important that andragogy does not become elevated, too quickly, to the status of a 'model of learning' but rather that it is acknowledged as *prescription* for learning practices.

Returning to the concept of lifelong education, it may be seen that the 'romantic' approach to education may be the most appropriate model for fostering such a development. Romantic educational practices involve negotiation and attention to personal needs and wants. They also place much of the responsibility for learning firmly with the learner. Indeed Rogers (1983) argues that it is not possible to teach anyone anything: they can only be helped to learn. Thus personal responsibility in the learning process is not only advisable but an essential component. An appreciation of the romantic curriculum can enable nurse tutors, students and clinical practitioners to prepare themselves for lifelong learning.

On the other hand, there is also a clear place for the 'classical' approach. While it has been argued here that the two approaches begin from different theoretical positions, there is no reason why both classical and romantic approaches cannot be used. There are aspects of the nursing curriculum which need to be 'taught', in the sense of passing on of concrete knowledge and skills. All nurses need a sound knowledge and skills base from which to work and there may be sound economic reasons why, in the initial stages of nurse education, the 'classical' approach can be useful. If nurses are 'taught' certain basic approaches to learning, ways of developing theories, methods of using learning resources (books, articles, videos, libraries, bibliographies, etc.), then they may later move on to a more 'romantic' approach, where they can use those basic learning skills efficiently and effectively.

The suggestion here is that learners begin with the classical approach to the curriculum and move towards the romantic approach as a means of working within the lifelong education model (Figure 3.5). In this way, there is a move from initial dependence on tutorial staff to an increasing state of independence and self-motivation. Linked to this educational process is the fact of clinical experience. As we have seen in the lifelong learning model, both educational and clinical processes go hand in hand. A valuable method of ensuring that they do is through the use of experiential learning.

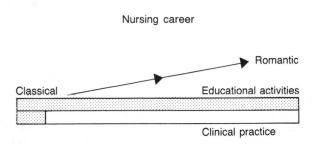

Nursing career

Romantic

Classical                    Educational activities

Clinical practice

**Figure 3.5**   Linking lifelong education with the classical/romantic curriculum

## Experiential learning

Experiential learning is learning through direct experience. It is 'personal' learning and, as such, has much in common with the concepts contained within the idea of the romantic curriculum. Experiential learning is most often linked with the learning of interpersonal skills – listening, counselling, talking to others, managing other people's distress and so forth (Kagan et al., 1986; Burnard, 1990b; Heron, 1973). It does, however, also have much wider application. The experiential learning cycle (Figure 3.6) can be used to 'process' any practical experience.

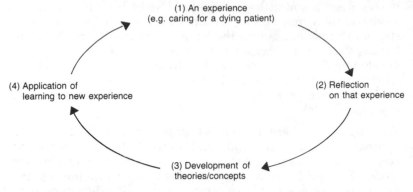

**Figure 3.6**  The experiential learning cycle

The experiential learning cycle involves four stages. Stage one is the experience itself (caring for a dying patient, talking to relatives, working in theatre and so forth). Stage two involves the process of quietly reflecting on that experience and attempting to recall all or most aspects of it, good and bad. This reflective period is, perhaps, the most important stage in the cycle. It is tempting to think that a person always learns from experience. The fact is, perhaps, that a person only learns from experience if that experience is reflected upon. Experience that just 'happens' is rarely of any lasting value, it goes by unnoticed and unremarked.

In stage three of the cycle, new learning in the form of theories and concepts is drawn out of the experience. Once the reflective period has taken place, the individual 'makes sense' of his experience and relates it to past experience and to the literature and research on the topic. Again, this period of 'making sense' is very important. It is insufficient merely to acknowledge that an experience has occurred; the full implications of that experience need to be explored if new learning is to take place.

In stage four, that new learning is applied in practice. In the context of nursing, this application will usually be in the clinical situation. Table 3.2 offers an example of the experiential learning cycle in use. In this example, practical nursing experience has been followed by reflection on that experience. Out of that reflective process has evolved a variety of theoretical and conceptual issues which have led the nurse to further study. New learning has then been carried over into practical experience and thus the

*Stage One: An Experience:*
Caring for a dying patient

*Stage Two: Reflection on that Experience:*
Personal involvement/emotion
Consideration of patient's physical needs
Difficulty in *talking* to patient
Patient's spiritual needs?
Patient's knowledge about their own predicament
My knowledge of the patient
My *own* thoughts about dying
My relationship wtih other staff
Pain management, etc.

*Stage Three: Development of Theories/Concepts:*
Need for *personal* interpersonal skills training
Stages of dying? Kubler-Ross?
Facing death and spiritual needs: is there a direct relationship? Check literature, etc.

*Stage Four: Application of Learning to New Experience:*
Caring, more sensitively, more knowledgeably

**Table 3.2**  An example of the experiential learning cycle in use

cycle has been continued. Throughout the process, experience leads to new knowledge and that new knowledge informs practice.

A major factor in the use of the experiential learning cycle is the development of the self-reflective ability used in stage two of the cycle. Much of life is lived without noticing what is being thought or felt. For the experiential learning cycle to work it is required that individuals notice themselves and become more aware of what they are doing. Such awareness takes concentration and patience but once mastered can become a useful tool for living. It can be enhanced through practices such as meditation and co-counselling (Bond, 1986; Burnard, 1985), both of which improve the ability to concentrate and to pay attention. Courses in these methods are frequently offered by extra-mural departments of colleges and universities.

Experiential and reflective learning methods have been incorporated into many college nursing programmes. However, they need to be used judiciously. In a study of nurse teachers' and nurse educators' perceptions of experiential learning, Burnard found that while most agreed that experiential learning methods enhanced self-awareness and encouraged the development of interpersonal skills, many student nurses found the methods that involved a high level of participation and possible self-disclosure embarrassing to take part in (Burnard, 1991). In particular, most of the students found role play and the use of 'icebreaker' exercises particularly difficult to work with. In another study of nurse teachers and nursing students, Burnard and Morrison (1992) found that while many nurse educators thought it essential to use 'student-centred' approaches to learning and teaching, many students looked for more direction and information-giving from teachers. It was as though the teachers favoured a 'student-centred' approach while the students preferred a 'teacher-centred' approach. If nurse educators really do want to keep in mind the needs and wants of their students it would seem that they must *listen* to those students. The students may well be telling the teachers what sort of educational experiences they want.

Thus the means by which the nurse may 'take every reasonable opportunity to maintain and improve professional knowledge and competence' may be summarised as follows. There should be an appreciation the need for lifelong education by both nurse educators and by individual practitioners. Responsibility for learning needs should be taken by all nurses once they have established basic knowledge and skills. There may need to be a gradual move from a 'classical' curriculum towards a 'romantic' curriculum. Again, the individual nurse can gain much from considering the principles of such a curriculum. All nurses need to develop a reflective ability that makes them aware of their own thoughts, feelings and actions. Such reflection can be an important method of modifying future nursing practice. A person cannot do anything about himself until he knows something about himself. Such knowledge can come through regular use of the experiential learning cycle. Thus professional knowledge and competence starts with personal knowledge and competence. This theme is developed further in the next chapter. Before that, however, it is necessary to review, briefly, the *actual* changes that have occurred in professional nurse education in the UK in the past few years.

## Changes in nursing education

In order to assess the degree to which the ideas in this chapter can or cannot be put into operation, it is necessary to identify the changes that have taken place in nurse education in the past few years. Clearly, the most important change has been that brought about by Project 2000.

In 1986 the UKCC issued a document entitled *Project 2000: A New Preparation for Practice*. This was the result of the deliberations of a working group set up by the UKCC which contained representatives of the various disciplines within nursing, of further and higher education and from the UKCC and the four National Boards. During the deliberations of this group members consulted widely with the profession by issuing papers on specific topics and by conducting 'road shows'. Feedback from both these activities was incorporated into a document which went out for final consultation to the profession. The final recommendations, when issued, were seen to be a joint exercise between the five statutory bodies – the UKCC and the four National Boards – and as such were presented to representatives of Government from England, Scotland, Wales and Northern Ireland.

The changes brought about by Project 2000 can be broadly summarised as follows.

In order to produce an educated individual able to react to rapidly changing health care needs, a 'knowledgeable doer', and to reduce duplication in training programmes as well as to reduce waste from nurse training, the following were proposed:

## One level of qualified (registered) nurse

In order to achieve this, state enrolled nurse training was to be discontinued and those enrolled nurses who so wished and were able to do so, were to be offered 'conversion' courses to enable them to reach registration status. In recent months, the UKCC has issued a directive that allows registered nurses to call themselves 'RNs' (registered nurses) whatever their original registration designation was. Thus RGNs, RMNs, RSCNs and RNMHs can all use the designation registered nurse. Predictably, not all registered nurses have wanted to undergo this change in title and the UKCC has added a proviso that those registered nurses who wish to may continue to use their original designations.

## Change in the emphasis of nursing education

In future the emphasis was to be rooted in health not disease, with an increased emphasis on health education and preventive care. It was also recommended that the registered nurse be prepared to function equally well outside as well as inside institutions.

## Change in the pattern of nursing education

The proposal was for a 'common foundation programme' lasting two years. This programme was to contain foundation knowledge in the biological and behavioural sciences, interpersonal and communication skills, fundamental nursing theory and practice with experience in a wide range of settings, both within hospitals and in non-institutional settings. Following successful completion of the foundation programme, students would then be able to proceed to a 'branch programme' in one of four areas: care of the adult, care of the child, care of the mentally handicapped or mental health nursing. The proposal was that the branch programme would last one year. These times were later altered as a result of professional pressure so that the final proposal is for a common foundation programme of 18 months followed by a further 18 months in one of the branch programmes.

A letter to the Statutory Bodies was issued by the Government on 10 May 1989 to deal with some of the matters not clarified in the letter of 20 May 1988. These are as follows:

### Student service contribution

In order to assist in manpower planning the Government requires that students contribute not less than 1000 hours of rostered service during the three-year programme and that this should normally be in the third year.

### All-graduate teaching force

Although the Government realises that an increasing proportion of the profession and its teaching staff hold degrees it does not consider that other non-graduate teaching staff should be excluded. As a result of the recommendation that nurse teachers should also be graduates, many non-graduate nurse teachers have begun or completed degrees in nursing. Many have taken the graduate route through Master's degree courses which have allowed them to register as postgraduate students by virtue of their professional experience and their previous qualifications. This has led to a debate about the degree to which the various academic levels in nursing 'fit' together (Davis and Burnard, 1992). It is no longer always clear exactly what the differences are between

Bachelor's and Master's degrees although, by virtue of their existence at all, there *should* be differences between them.

## Midwifery education and training

The Government expressed a welcome for the expansion of direct midwifery education and training and accepted that this should be broadly along the same lines as that for nurses in terms of supernumerary status and rostered service contribution. Shared learning with nursing students was seen as desirable, both to facilitate subsequent collaborative professional working and to maximise the use of scarce educational resources.

Project 2000 courses have been linked to higher education institutions and concluded at diploma level which has also put pressure on teaching staff to become graduates.

## Entry to nursing

The Government, while recognising steps were being taken to widen the entry-gate to nursing, wished to see greater practical evidence of the profession accepting vocational qualifications as satisfying the UKCC's entry requirements for nursing, this being particularly relevant for the support worker. In addition the Government expressed the hope that access courses to nursing would be developed in line with those established for access to higher education.

Finally, that while not directly the responsibility of the statutory bodies, efforts should be made to reduce the rigidity regarding admission criteria demonstrated by some schools and colleges of nursing. This has been enhanced by the recognition of life experience and work in clinical areas as often compensatory for formal educational qualifications.

## Support worker

This grade has the potential for attracting both young and mature entrants to the caring role and progress to an appropriate NCVQ level vocational qualification should permit access to nurse training programmes. This would also be in accordance with the Government's views on 'links and ladders' between various vocational qualifications.

The Government expressed dissatisfaction with the title 'support worker' for those working within the health care setting and wondered if 'health care assistant' would be more suitable; this is the title that has been adopted.

## Enrolled nurse training

The Government felt that, providing the steps regarding access and the support worker were taken, then enrolled nurse training could cease within the next five years. However where Project 2000 was implemented locally then EN training should be discontinued as part of the implementation process. Greater flexibility in enrolled nurse conversion courses was sought by Government and their continued contribution to care acknowledged. Various *open learning* courses have been developed to enable enrolled nurses to become registered nurses, including one sponsored and developed by the *Nursing Times*. However, a frequent matter of debate in the nursing journals is the fact that many enrolled nurses have found it difficult to get places on conversion courses.

## Conclusion

What remains less clear is the degree to which some of the principles outlined in this chapter will be affected by the changes brought about by Project 2000. Although Project 2000 courses have meant more autonomy for students in some respects, in others, the position is less clear. Larger groups of students tend to mean that lecturers return to a 'lecture' approach to education. The small group work that might be developed to encourage autonomy in learning might be lost if student groups continue to grow and little further investment is made in financing more lecturing posts. The next few years should clarify the degree to which the profession really is committed to the development of autonomous, reflective and critical thinkers and the degree to which student nurse education returns to a more prescriptive and 'classical' style. At the time of writing, the Government is questioning the cost of implementing the PREPP recommendations.

## Questions for reflection and discussion

1. To what degree are *you* up to date in your nursing knowledge?
2. Are the nurses that you know 'reflective practitioners'?

# References

Atwood AH (1979) The mentor in clinical practice. *Nursing Outlook* **27**: 714–717.

Bond M (1986) *Stress and Self-Awareness: a Guide for Nurses.* London: Heinemann.

Brookfield SD (1987) *Developing Critical Thinkers: Challenging Adults to Explore Alternative Ways of Thinking and Acting.* Milton Keynes: Open University Press.

Brown BJ (1984) The dean as mentor. *Nursing Health Care* **5**(2) 88–91.

Burnard P (1985) Future imperfect? *Senior Nurse* **2**(1): 8–10.

Burnard P (1987) Self and peer assessment. *Senior Nurse* **6**(5): 16–17.

Burnard P (1989) The role of mentor. *Journal of District Nursing* **8**(3): 8–10.

Burnard P (1990) Is anyone here a mentor? *Nursing Standard* **4**(37): 46.

Burnard P (1990) *Learning Human Skills: an Experiential Guide for Nurses.* Oxford: Butterworth-Heinemann.

Burnard P (1991) *Experiential Learning in Action.* Aldershot: Avebury.

Burnard P and Morrison P (1992) Students' and lecturers' preferred teaching strategies. *International Journal of Nursing Studies* **29**(4): 345–353.

Burton A (1977) The mentoring dynamic in the therapeutic transformation. *The American Journal of Psychoanalysis* **37**: 115–122.

Darling LAW (1984) What do nurses want in a mentor? *The Journal of Nursing Administration* **October**: 42–44.

Davis BD and Burnard P (1992) Academic levels in nursing. *Journal of Advanced Nursing* **17**: 1395–1400.

Donovan J (1990) The concept and role of mentor. *Nurse Education Today* **10**: 294–298.

Freire P (1980) *Cultural Action for Freedom.* Harmondsworth: Penguin.

Heron J (1973) *Experiential Training Techniques.* Human Potential Research Project. Guildford: University of Surrey.

Jarvis P (1983a) *The Theory and Practice of Adult and Continuing Education.* London: Croom Helm.

Jarvis P (1983b) *The Sociology of Adult and Continuing Education.* London: Croom Helm.

Kagan C, et al. (1986) *Interpersonal Skills Training for Nurses: an Experiential Approach.* London: Harper and Row.

Kilty J (1981) *Self and Peer Assessment.* Human Potential Research Project. Guildford: University of Surrey.

Knowles M (1981) *The Adult Learner: a Neglected Species* (2nd edition). Texas: Gulf.

Lawton D (1973) *Social Change, Educational Theory and Curriculum Planning.* London: Hodder and Stoughton.

Peters RS (1969) *Ethics and Education.* London: Allen and Unwin.

Pirsig R (1976) *Zen and the Art of Motorcycle Maintenance.* London: Arrow.

Rogers C-R (1983) *Freedom to Learn for the Eighties.* Columbus, Ohio: Merrill.

UKCC (1986) *Project 2000.* London: United Kingdom Central Council for Nursing Midwifery and Health Visiting.

Whitehead AN (1932) *The Aims of Education.* London: Benn.

# CHAPTER 4

# Knowing your Limitations

*Acknowledge any limitations in your knowledge and competence and decline any duties or responsibilities unless able to perform them in a safe and skilled manner.*

Nurses must know their limits: they must have a firm understanding of what they know and what they do not know, what skills they have and what skills they lack. In order to appreciate limits it is necessary to develop self-awareness. But what is self-awareness and how can it be developed? In order to answer these questions it may be helpful to identify those aspects that go to make up a concept of self.

Developing the work of Carl Jung (1983), five aspects of the self may be identified: sensing, thinking, feeling, intuiting and body experience.

These five aspects of the self will now be considered and methods identified for developing awareness in each of them. It should be acknowledged that this is only one way of analysing the concept of self. The concept is a complicated one, which has been debated by philosophers, theologians, psychologists and sociologists for centuries. What is important, here, is that a concrete and usable concept of self may be useful in nursing. For other concepts and discussions of the question of self, the reader is referred to Williams (1973), Canfield and Wells (1976), Rogers (1951) and Macquarrie (1973).

The first four domains of the self, identified above, refer to internal psychological aspects. Jung summarises, concisely, the function of each of these aspects:

The essential function of sensation is to establish that something exists, thinking tells us what it means, feeling what its value is and intuition surmises whence it comes and wither it goes. (Jung, 1983, p. 144)

## Sensing

The first aspect, then, is sensation. It is arguable that everything that is thought about or felt is experienced first through one or more of the five special senses: hearing, seeing, tasting, touching and smelling, of which the first two are perhaps the most highly developed. In order that the individual can make sense of the world at all, that world must first be experienced via the senses.

It is easy, however, for attention to the senses to be lost. Very often a person is so distracted by their thoughts and feelings that they fail to pay full attention to what they see or hear. In this way the person fails to take full advantage of an educational encounter or alternatively a considerable amount of a patient's communication is lost. In order to appreciate fully the inputs that are being received through the senses, a person must concentrate on them. A simple experiment may serve to drive this point home. Stop reading this book for a moment and pay close attention to what you can hear around you. As you do so, you will suddenly notice how much auditory input has been filtered out prior to undertaking the experiment.

Such filtering out is essential at times but at others it is necessary to resist this shutting off process and pay close attention to what is going on around you. Part of becoming more self-aware is the process of 'noticing': simply paying attention to what is being seen and heard. The development of such attention can help to ensure greater accuracy of reporting, greater observational skills and a greater resistance to making snap judgments and evaluations. The person who pays conscious attention to what they are seeing or hearing gathers accurate data and therefore is in a better position to make considered judgments. Such a position is in line with the Code of Conduct's requirement that nurses acknowledge their limitations of competence.

## Thinking

Once information enters through one of the senses, it is thought about. Thinking, here, refers to the processes of puzzling, pondering, analysing and criticising. It is essential that the person reflects upon what they know, on whether or not what they know is accurate and what they need to develop in terms of knowledge. In this sense, it is necessary to develop a continuous and consistent ability to be critical: to question regularly what is held to be true. This is not a comfortable process! It is sometimes far easier to hang on to an old set of beliefs that has been useful in the past than to question the validity of those beliefs. It is far less comfortable still, to adopt Marx's favourite maxim 'doubt everything' (Singer, 1980).

This inner reflection on knowledge and upon its validity and present-day utility value is again part of the requirement being proposed by the Code of Conduct. To acknowledge limitations and to refuse to accept certain delegated functions is first to have pondered upon one's own knowledge and skills base.

## Feelings

The next aspect of the self is feelings. The term feelings, here, refers to the whole spectrum of emotions that may be felt, ranging on the one hand, from elation to, on the other, profound depression. What is important is that the individual learns to develop the ability to identify and acknowledge her feelings in a given situation. In nursing it is often far easier (and sometimes encouraged) either to ignore or rationalise feelings as they occur in day-to-day practice and even to pretend that they just do not exist. This is evident in the image of the nurse as an implacable, objective carer who has somehow learned to detach herself from the issue of emotion. Quite how this image has arisen over the years is unclear but the effects of such a situation are well documented by Bond (1986). She points out that consistent bottling up of emotion can lead to frustration, anxiety and to burnout – total disenchantment with the process of nursing and caring.

Heron (1977) notes that, among other things, the bottling up of feelings in this way can lead to:

1. physical tension, with resultant muscular tension and postural problems,
2. mental blocks and the inability to concentrate and make decisions,
3. emotional numbness: inability to express any sort of positive feelings – love, caring, affection and so forth,
4. emotional outbursts, where the bottled up emotion suddenly rushes to the surface and manifests itself in outbursts of tears of anger.

Heron offers a comprehensive account of how emotions become bottled up through the process of living and how emotional release can lead to clearer thinking and more rational decision-making.

To attempt to bottle up feelings in this way is also a strategy that rarely works completely, as emotional feelings are usually 'given away' by the person's facial expression, tone of voice, choice of words, use of metaphors, hand gestures and so forth (Argyle, 1976; Bandler and Grinder, 1982). We are always communicating. Even when we think that we have successfully camouflaged our feelings, they tend to leak out! What is being advocated here, is not that nurses disclose all their feelings to patients but that it is helpful to all relationships if feelings can be identified by the individual as they occur. If such identification can take place and the person, through reflection, can acknowledge how she feels, then the individual can choose whether to express her feelings, ignore them, or deal with them later. If no such identification of feelings occurs, no such range of choices exists. If, through acting in this reflective way, the individual decides to deal with her feelings later, a number of other options become available. At some time later, those feelings can be talked through with a friend or a colleague. Alternatively, a more structured approach such as co-counselling can be used (Heron, 1974, 1978).

## Co-counselling

Co-counselling courses are offered by a number of extra-mural departments of universities and by many further and higher education departments of colleges. Co-counselling has also been advocated as a peer support strategy in nurse education (Kilty, 1983). In essence, the method requires that two people, trained in co-counselling, meet for an allotted time. They then spend half of that time in the role of counsellor to the other's role of client. They then switch roles for the other half of the time. In this way, both people get equal amounts of time to talk through problems, express pent up feelings and to design new coping strategies. It is important to note, however, that in co-counselling, the role of 'client' is the most important one and the person occupying the role of 'counsellor' does not counsel in the traditional sense of the word. They do not offer advice nor make suggestions as to how the other person may 'put her life right'. Instead they act more as a 'sounding board' for the client, who, in this relationship, soon learns to 'counsel herself'. In this sense, then, the client in the co-counselling relationship retains autonomy and does not become dependent on the counsellor.

Other options available to the person who decides to deal with emotions later include the use of meditation (Le Shan, 1974; Hewitt, 1978), and the transmutation of strong emotion through sport or exercise. A further range of methods for coping with emotions is offered by Bond (1986) and with particular reference to nurses. Decisions about how a particular individual copes with stress are often matters of personal preference, pesonality type and practical considerations such as time and resources. It is remarkable, however, how frequently the nurse 'puts off' the process of practically dealing with stress, claiming to be 'too busy'!

Given the stressful nature of nursing and the fact that even very junior nurses are frequently called upon to look after people in particularly difficult circumstances, it would seem reasonable to suggest that the domain of feelings needs addressing more fully in both clinical and educational circles. The profession cannot afford to carry on as though nurses were somehow uninvolved emotionally. Human suffering always calls for involvement and involvement in the human condition always concerns feelings. To ignore the domain of feelings in nurses is to ignore an important part of what it means to be a human being.

## Intuition

The fourth aspect of the self is the intuitive domain. Intuition refers to a hunch or notion that may occur apparently independently of the senses. It is as if we know something to be the case without our necessarily having confirming evidence for it. Such intuition may be explained away in terms of some elaborate cognitive process that is yet to be understood, or it may be thought of as some sort of unconscious process. For others, it has mystical connotations. However it is explained and whatever theories are offered for it, it does appear to be an important phenomenon. Indeed, the counsellor and therapist Carl Rogers argued that he was functioning at his most therapeutically when he paid attention to and acted upon his intuitive feelings during a counselling session (Rogers, 1967). In the nursing field, Benner (1984) argues from her research that very skilled nursing practitioners often make decisions about nursing intervention intuitively.

The argument here is that the nurse needs to pay attention to this intuitive aspect as an important part of self-awareness. It is these sudden intuitive ideas that occur during conversations with patients that can lead to useful problem-solving and important changes in care. This aspect of care might be called the 'artistic' side as compared to the 'scientific' side, which tends to remain firmly rooted in the cognitive and rational domain. Equally important, however, is the need to balance such intuition with a calm, rational and logical approach to work and care. Just as we cannot always deliver thorough and systematic care through appeal only to logic and science, neither can we rely only on intuition. Indeed, Jung (1983) argued that the self-aware person was the one who could balance all four aspects of mind: thinking, feeling, sensing and intuiting – for all are important.

## Body experience

A final aspect of self is body experience. It is possible to talk about the body as if it were somehow detached from the rest of the person. Thus it is not uncommon to hear people use expressions such as 'I don't like my body' or 'I'm not happy with my body', as though it were something of an appendage! To talk of a self-concept must be to include a bodily sense of self. Thus part of developing self-awareness is developing an accurate body image and perhaps a sense of responsibility for the body. In recent years, nurses have become increasingly aware of the part they play in acting as positive role-models in the campaign against smoking. It is notable that the Royal College of Nursing has a definite no-smoking policy regarding its premises. It would appear, then, that in matters of physical health and appearance, nurses should also pay attention to how they present themselves to the public. Christine Hancock makes this point rather forcibly when she says that:

> We are often saying publicly we claim to believe in health but really we like ill health, sickness and early death. (Hancock, 1987, p. 9)

She goes on to argue that nurses must improve their presentation of self to the public. Part of this process begins with the individual's awareness of their own body, its appearance and its capabilities. Again, this is in keeping with the fourth statement of the Code of Conduct. Part of competence and appreciating limits is an awareness of one's own physical strength (or lack of it), agility and ability to exercise psychomotor dexterity.

Further, the more psychological aspects of self are perhaps mediated by our physical sense of self. Thus our internal self-image is usually improved by a confident and healthy external presentation. There are, of course, numerous methods of increasing the physical sense of well-being, ranging from exercise and diet to specific sporting and recreational activities.

This, then, is an approach to understanding the concepts of self and self-awareness. Such awareness is a necessary prerequisite of any decision-making about whether or not to accept delegated instructions in nursing practice. Once we are aware of our abilities and deficits, we are in a position to do something about them. Without such awareness, we are 'blind' and because of that blindness, probably less effective in our delivery of care.

Once limitations have been discovered, the next stage is to rectify them. This is where the notion of self-directed learning alluded to in the previous chapter is particularly appropriate. Malcolm Knowles (1975) advocates the use of personal learning contracts. Such a contract can be designed by an individual nurse in co-operation with a nurse tutor or a lecturer. Alternatively, the contract can be written out for its own sake as a method of clarifying learning objectives and methods of evaluation. Thirdly, it can be used in the clinical setting as part of a learning programme or as an aspect of staff development. Table 4.1 is an example of a learning contract. Such a contract identifies learning objectives, learning

| Learning contract | | | |
|---|---|---|---|
| Name: John Doe | Learning project: applying the nursing process in psychiatric nursing | | |
| 1 Learning objectives | 2 Learning resources and strategies | 3 Evidence of accomplishment | 4 Criteria and means of validating evidence |
| 1 To define the nursing process | – the library<br>– the School of Nursing<br>– nursing journals | A short essay on the nursing process | Presentation of the essay at a ward meeting attended by a clinical teacher |
| 2 To use the nursing process in planning the care of two patients | – the charge nurse<br>– the clinical teacher<br>– books on the subject | Two care plans written out in the patients' notes | Rating of the care plans by two peers and by the clinical teacher and charge nurse |

**Table 4.1** An example of a learning contract

C

resources and evaluation methods in such a way as to ensure that a thorough educational experience is undertaken.

By regular use of a learning contract and through maintenance and development of self-awareness, the nurse can monitor her own performance in terms of statement four of the Code of Conduct. Limitations of competence can be the basis from which to move forward and to develop an ever-widening range of skills and knowledge. Such development is in keeping with present-day educational theory which stresses the need for continuing and lifelong education (Jarvis, 1983). No longer can basic nurse training be expected to serve the nurse throughout her career nor can nurse education remain an impartial knowledge-based process. Today it is vital that self-knowledge be incorporated into this lifelong process of learning to nurse.

## Questions for reflection and discussion

1. Is it possible to become self-aware?
2. What are the pros and cons of learning contracts?

## References

Argyle M (1976) *The Psychology of Interpersonal Behaviour*. Harmondsworth: Penguin.
Bander R and Grinder J (1982) *Reframing: Neuro-Linguistic Programming and the Transformation of Meaning*. Moab, Utah: Real People Press.
Benner P (1984) *From Novice to Expert: Excellence and Power in Clinical Nursing Practice*. Menlo Park, California: Addison–Wesley.
Bond M (1986) *Stress and Self-Awareness: a Guide for Nurses*. London: Heinemann.
Canfield J and Wells HC (1976) *100 Ways to Enhance Self-Concept in the Classroom*. Englewood Cliffs, New Jersey; Prentice Hall.
Hancock C (1987) Generally speaking. *Senior Nurse* 6(4): 8–9.
Heron J (1974) *Reciprocal Counselling Manual*. Human Potential Research Project. Guildford: University of Surrey.
Heron J (1977) *Catharsis in Human Development*. Human Potential Research Project. Guildford: University of Surrey.
Heron J (1978) *Co-Counsellor's Teacher's Manual*. Human Potential Research Project. Guildford: University of Surrey.
Hewitt J (1978) *Meditation*. Sevenoaks, Kent: Hodder and Stoughton.
Jarvis P (1983) *The Theory and Practice of Adult and Continuing Education*. London: Croom Helm.
Jung CG (1983) *Selected Writings* (A Storr, ed). London: Pan.
Kilty J (1983) *Experiential Learning*. Human Potential Research Project. Guildford: University of Surrey.

Knowles M (1975) *Self-Directed Learning: A Guide for Learners and Teachers.* New York: Cambridge.
Le Shan M.(1974) *How to Meditate.* Wellingborough: Turnstone Press.
Macquarrie J (1973) *Existentialism.* Harmondsworth: Penguin.
Rogers CR (1951) *Client-Centred Counselling.* London: Constable.
Rogers CR (1967) *On Becoming a Person.* London: Constable.
Singer P (1980) *Marx.* Oxford: Oxford University Press.
Williams B (1973) *The Problem of Self.* Cambridge: Cambridge University Press.

**CHAPTER 5**

# Working with Patients, Clients and Families

*Work in an open and co-operative manner with patients, clients and their families; foster their independence and recognise and respect their involvement in the planning and delivery of care.*

There is a real danger that when a person becomes a patient the health care team feels that they 'possess' that individual and that as a patient the person has to surrender all 'rights' to them. This is not so: the patient or, if the patient is unable to express an opinion by reason of illness or handicap, a relative or guardian, has the right to information regarding treatment and care; to understand the prognosis; to appreciate possible side-effects of treatment and to be made aware of alternative strategies. When this information has been made available then a decision to accept the treatment and care offered or to decline it is still the prerogative of the patient.

## Patients' rights

The American Hospital Association has formulated a Patient's Bill of Rights (1973) reproduced below.

1. The patient has the right to considerate and respectful care.

2. The patient has the right to obtain from his physician complete current information concerning his diagnosis, treatment and prognosis in terms the patient can reasonably be expected to understand. When it is not medically advisable to give such information to the patient, the information should be made available to an appropriate person on his behalf. He has the right to know, by name, the physician responsible for co-ordinating his care.

3. The patient has the right to receive from his physician information necessary to give informed consent prior to the start of any procedure and/or treatment. Except in emergencies, such information for informed consent should include but not necessarily be limited to the specific procedure and/or treatment, the medically significant risks involved and the probable duration of incapacitation. Where medically significant alternatives for care or treatment exist, or where the patient requests information concerning medical alternatives, the patient has the right to such information. The patient also has the right to know the name of the person responsible for the procedures or treatment.

4. The patient has the right to refuse treatment to the extent permitted by law, and to be informed of the medical consequences of his action.

5. The patient has the right to every consideration of his privacy concerning his own medical care programme. Case discussion, consultation, examination and treatment are confidential and should be conducted discreetly. Those not directly involved in his care must have the permission of the patient to be present.

6. The patient has the right to expect that all communications and records pertaining to his care should be treated as confidential.

7. The patient has the right to expect that within its capacity a hospital must make reasonable response to the request by a patient for services. The hospital must provide evaluation, service and/or referral as indicated by the urgency of the case. When medically permissible a patient may be transferred to another facility only after he has received complete information and full explanation concerning the need for and alternatives to such a transfer. The institution to which the patient is to be transferred must first have accepted the patient for transfer.

8. The patient has the right to obtain information as to any relationship of his hospital to other health care and educational institutions insofar as his care is concerned. The patient has the right to obtain information as to the existence of any professional relationship among individuals, by name, who are treating him.

9. The patient has the right to be advised if the hospital proposes to engage in or perform human experimentation affecting his care or treatment. The patient has the right to refuse to participate in such research projects.

10. The patient has the right to expect reasonable continuity of care. He has the right to know in advance what appointment times and physicians are available and where. The patient has the right

to expect that the hospital will provide a mechanism whereby he is informed by his physician or a delegate of the physician of his continuing health care requirements following discharge.

11. The patient has the right to examine and receive an explanation of his bill regardless of the source of payment.

12. The patient has the right to know what hospital rules and regulations apply to his conduct as a patient.

This Bill makes it quite explicit that the patient has to be considered as an equal part of the health care team concerned with his welfare, and although it refers to hospital patients the principles can and should also be applied to patients and clients receiving care in the community.

Many health care professionals pay lipservice to these rights but still feel that because of their position and superior knowledge and/or skill their views should carry more weight. The problem of paternalism or perhaps more accurately parentalism is ever-present in the health care setting. There is an implicit expectation among most health care professionals that the patient or client, by entering the health care institution, has surrendered all powers of intellect and has become in effect 'a little child'. Tied in with this is the somewhat Victorian attitude that 'children should be seen and not heard', hence the all-too-frequent complaint made by patients that the doctors or nurses not only did not explain the situation to them or consult them, but also in many cases they talked over them as if they did not exist. Linked with this approach is the view that the professional must know what is best for the patient or client and therefore should be obeyed. Such an approach is deeply resented by many patients who ask, quite rightly, 'whose life it?' Unfortunately, many patients lack the confidence or the skills of assertiveness to question doctors' decisions or to disagree with them. Often quiet compliance is the unhappy position adopted by many people when they become patients.

Remaining open and co-operative means being able to listen to the patients' or clients' expressed wants and needs. Also, as the second half of this item suggests, it also means encouraging independence. All of these ideas are recognised in contemporary approaches to nursing (Robinson and Vaughan, 1992) – particularly in the fields of primary nursing and client-centred care.

The notion of remaining open also involves appreciating the principles of client-centred communication. Carl Rogers (1967, 1983), father of client-centred counselling, developed a style of relating to others which involved the 'professional' in 'staying out of the client's way'. He suggested that far from advising and telling people what to do or to think, a more appropriate approach was to enable them to identify their own problems and to select their own solutions. The client-centred counselling that he developed involved the counsellor in a process in which the counsellor acted as a 'sounding board' for the client. The counsellor listened while the client talked and at no time did the counsellor become prescriptive. All of this was based on the premise that it is, in the end, impossible for one person to *decide* for another. In the end, we are free both to make life choices and also *have* to make such choices. The philosophical roots of such an approach lie in existential philosophy (Sartre, 1955). The approach has been described in detail elsewhere (Tschudin, 1991; Burnard, 1989). The client-centred approach to remaining open to the client's wants and needs has also been incorporated into nursing – particularly in the form of Orem's self-care model – and in primary nursing, itself, which views nursing as a *co-operative* venture in which the patient or client is encouraged to make decisions about both his nursing and his life (Robinson and Vaughan, 1992).

Client-centred counselling, itself, is also a means of practising the ideals laid down in this item of the Code. The nurse who is client-centred allows the patient to express her anxieties, fears and worries and helps her to find her own way through them via supportive and caring intervention. This is not to say that the nurse will no longer be called upon to advise on specific nursing and medical issues but that, in the domain of personal and emotional issues, the client is always the 'expert'. There are, however, limits to the client-centred approach and one area in which such limits may be evident is in the field of AIDS counselling. Nurses will find themselves increasingly being called upon to advise and help in this difficult field.

## AIDS counselling

AIDS, as everyone will now be aware, is one of the most serious diseases to threaten the world. Co-operation in this field is paramount if some degree of control of the spread of the disease is to be achieved. Those who receive AIDS counselling are not a homogeneous group. A list of the people who are likely to require counselling in this field is offered by Bor (1991):

1. Clients who have concerns or queries about AIDS, regardless of their clinical status.

2. Clients who are referred for the human immunodeficiency virus (HIV) antibody test.
3. Clients who are HIV antibody negative but who continue to present with AIDS-related worries.
4. Clients who are HIV antibody positive and symptomless.
5. Clients who are HIV antibody positive and who are becoming unwell.
6. Clients who have developed AIDS.
7. Clients who are being offered, or who are being considered for, antiviral treatments.
8. The sexual contacts, loved ones or family of any of the above, if the client has given his or her permission.
9. The close contacts of a deceased client, who may also later require bereavement counselling.
10. Staff with concerns about AIDS or those who are occupationally exposed to HIV (in conjunction with the occupational health department).

Given the diversity of this client group, it seems clear that different sorts of counselling skills and approaches are likely to be needed in AIDS counselling and that 'AIDS counselling' is not one particular entity. Bor concludes that 'there are many different counselling approaches and no evidence yet that one is better than another'.

For people who are substance abusers, Cook et al. (1988) suggest risk reduction counselling which includes:

1. Assisting the client to acknowledge the personal risks of HIV infection.
2. Explaining the range of changes that will reduce infection and transmission risks, addressing attitudinal and environmental obstacles (for example, feelings of having no control, resistance from partners) and rehearsing behaviours as needed.
3. Reinforcing changes in a way that helps the client to assume increasing control over health behaviours so that early accomplishments can be sustained and built upon.

Faltz (1989) offers the following guidelines for working with substance-abusing clients. Some of these may well be appropriate for other client groups.

1. Be willing to listen and encourage constructive expression of feelings.
2. Express caring and concern for the individual.
3. Hold the individual responsible for his actions.
4. Ensure consistent consequences for negative behaviours.

5. Talk to the individual about specific actions that are disruptive or disturbing.
6. Do not compromise your own values or expectations.
7. Communicate your plan of action to other staff members or professionals working with the client.
8. Monitor your own reactions to the client.

A wide range of other sorts of clients have been discussed in the AIDS counselling literature including: 'The worried well' (Bor et al., 1989), those who want or need to keep their diagnosis secret (Bor et al., 1986b), the counselling of antenatal women (Miller and Bor, 1990), children (Miller et al., 1989), those with haemophilia (DiMarzo, 1989) and ethnic minorities (Fullilove, 1989). Another group that might ask for counselling are bisexual people. The Off Pink Publishing Collective (1988), having noted of the paucity of research into bisexuality, write:

> Up until now the fact that maybe over a third of the population has strong attractions to or sexual activities with both sexes has generally been ignored. Sexual self-identities have been seen as either heterosexual, or gay or lesbian. But in reality people are not in distinct groups. As far as disease transmission is concerned, it is actual behaviour rather than self-identity that counts and many self-identified heterosexuals and gay men and lesbians behave bisexually. Contrary to a frequent association of bisexuality with promiscuity, it is our experience that many self-identified bisexuals are recurrently celibate, and increasingly so as part of a safer sex life.

Review of the literature on AIDS, AIDS counselling and sexuality tends to confirm the view that while bisexual people are noted to be at risk, they are less widely written about than are gay or heterosexual people.

## Some issues for the person with HIV/AIDS

There are numerous psychosocial issues facing the person who is HIV positive or who has AIDS. Silven and Caldarola (1989) suggest that many gay people who develop AIDS still see themselves as being punished for being gay. This idea can be further fuelled by those without AIDS who continue to suggest that people with AIDS are 'immoral' or 'dirty' (Kitzinger, 1990). Also, the person who lives a gay lifestyle and who knows other people with AIDS may well find that they have to experience the death of friends and may suffer from 'survival guilt' if they outlive their friends (Silven and Caldarola, 1989).

Friends and families respond and react in various ways to the knowledge that one of them is HIV positive or has AIDS. Not all are supportive and sometimes the person with AIDS has to face rejection by those he or she has loved (Perry and Tross, 1984). This may be coupled with the fact that facing AIDS can lead to psychological problems and feelings of dispiritedness and meaninglessness (Silven and Caldarola, 1989).

Clearly, there is also a whole range of physical problems to face. The person who is HIV positive may become understandably obsessed with looking for signs of having AIDS. Once AIDS is diagnosed, the person has to make further adjustments to a wide range of physical and psychological symptoms. Nor need the process be insidious. AIDS dementia, for example, can have a rapid onset and the first signs may be decreasing mental ability, quickly followed by a range of physical symptoms (Dilley and Boccellari, 1989).

Much anxiety often surrounds the issue of whether or not to be AIDS tested. The HIV antibody test has been available to those who want it since October 1985 (in the UK) and most Western countries have introduced facilities for such testing. There are specific issues in counselling for the counsellor who faces a person who is unsure about whether or not to be tested. McCreaner (1989) identifies the aims of pre-test counselling as follows:

1. To ensure that any decision to take the test is fully informed and based on an understanding of the personal, medical, legal and social implications of a positive result. At one level, this is a mere practical application of the traditional medical ethic of informed consent to a procedure.
2. To provide the necessary preparation for those who will have to face the trauma of a positive result. Such preparation is vital in that patients who have been prepared for a positive result are able to face that result much more equably.
3. To provide the individual, whether he eventually elects not to be tested, or elects to be tested and is found positive or found to be negative, with necessary risk reduction information on the basis of which he can reduce the risk of either acquiring HIV infection or passing it on to others.

Green (1989) offers a comprehensive list of the issues that need to be covered by the AIDS counsellor who is offering post-test counselling and where the result of the test has been positive:

1. Break the news in a clear and sympathetic way.
2. Listen carefully to the patient's response and help him to talk through what it means to him.

3. Provide facts about HIV and AIDS.
4. Provide facts about transmission.
5. Provide information about infection control issues.
6. Find out about the patient's sex life.
7. Find out about his relationships.
8. Find out about any other risk factors, e.g. injecting drug user.
9. Help him to implement safer sex.
10. Help him to reduce other risk factors.
11. Help him to inform sexual partners.
12. Help him to deal with relationship issues.
13. Help him to arrange a social support network or to make the best use of the one he has.
14. Inform him about what hospital and voluntary services are available to help him, and how to access them.
15. Help him to decide who else he wishes to tell.
16. Encourage him to take positive steps to maintain and improve general health.
17. Organise further appointments with the counsellor, and with other health workers.
18. Make sure that he has adequate medical support and services.
19. Help him with practical problems such as housing, welfare benefits, etc.
20. Make sure that he knows how to reach the counsellor in case of difficulty and knows he is welcome to seek help from the counsellor.

## Working together

In this chapter we have briefly explored two ends of a spectrum of psychological interventions. On the one hand, we have discussed the client-centred approach to patient care. As we have seen, in this approach, the client is the 'expert'. At the other end of the scale, we have explored, also, a domain in which the nurse is likely to be called upon for advice and for very specific information. There are numerous nursing situations in between these two extremes in which the nurse will sometimes be listener and befriender, and also adviser, and someone who is able to supply accurate and up-to-date information. Part of the process of working with individuals and families is learning to negotiate *boundaries* between professional expertise and knowledge on the one hand, and personal freedom and autonomy on the other. In the end, nursing and patient relationships are *negotiated* out of the perceived needs of the client and the wider needs of the family and even of society at large. None of us lives in isolation: we need to consider both personal wants and needs, the needs of families and friends and also the needs of the general public whenever we plan nursing actions.

## Questions for reflection and discussion

1. To what degree was AIDS an important topic on *your* training syllabus?
2. Are *you* a client-centred practitioner?

### References

American Hospital Association (1973) *A Patient's Bill of Rights*. New York: AMA.

Bor R, Miller R and Perry L (1989a) Strategies for counselling the 'worried well' in relation to AIDS. *Journal of the Royal Society of Medicine* **23**: 218–220.

Bor R, Miller R and Salt H (1989b) Secrecy related problems in AIDS management. *Journal of the Royal College of Physicians* **23**: 264–267.

Bor R (1991) The ABC of AIDS counselling. *Nursing Times* **87**(1) 32–35.

Burnard P (1989) Existentialism as a theoretical basis for counselling in psychiatric nursing. *Archives of Psychiatric Nursing* **III**(3) 142–147.

Cook A, Fischer G and Jones E (1988) *Preventing AIDS Among Substance Abusers: A Training for Substance Abuse Treatment Counsellors*. Falls Church, VA: The Center for AIDS and Substance Abuse Training.

Dilley JW and Boccellari A (1989) Neuropsychiatric complications of HIV infection. In: Dilley JW, Pies C and Helquist M (eds) *Face to Face: A Guide to AIDS Counselling*. University of California, San Francisco, California: AIDS Health Project.

DiMarzo D (1989) Double jeopardy: haemophilia and HIV disease. In: Donoghue M, Stimson G and Dolan K (eds) Sexual behaviour of injecting drug users and associated risks of HIV infection for non-injecting sexual partners. *AIDS Care* **1**: 51–58.

Falz BG (1989) Strategies for working with substance abusing clients. In: Dilley JW, Pies C and Helquist M (eds) *Face to Face: A Guide to AIDS Counselling*. University of California, San Francisco: AIDS Health Project.

Fullilove MT (1989) Ethnic minorities, HIV disease and the growing underclass. In: Dilly JW, Pies C and Helquist M (eds) *Face to Face: A Guide to AIDS Counselling*. University of California, San Francisco, California: AIDS Health Project.

Green J (1989) Post-test counselling. In: Green J and McCreaner A (eds) *Counselling in HIV Infection and AIDS*. London: Blackwell.

Kitzinger J (1990) Audience understandings of AIDS media messages: a discussion of methods. *Sociology of Health and Illness* **12**(3) 319–335.

McCreaner A (1989) Pre-test counselling. In: Green J and McCreaner A (eds) *Counselling in HIV Infection and AIDS*. London: Blackwell.

Miller R and Bor R (1990) Counselling for HIV screening in women. In: Studd J (ed) *Progress in Obstetrics and Gynaecology*. Edinburgh: Churchill Livingstone.

Miller R, Goldman E and Bor R (1989) Counselling children and adults about AIDS/HIV. *Counselling Psychology Quarterly* **2**: 65–72.

Off Pink Publishing Collective (1988) *Bisexual Lives*. London: Off Pink Publishing Collective.

Perry S and Tross S (1984) *Psychiatric Problems of AIDS Inpatients at the New York Hospital: a Preliminary Report*. Public Health Reports **99**: 200–205.

Robinson K and Vaughan B (eds) (1992) *Knowledge for Nursing Practice*. Oxford: Butterworth-Heinemann.

Rogers CR (1967) *On Becoming a Person*. London: Constable.

Rogers CR (1983) *Freedom to Learn for the Eighties*. Columbus, Ohio: Merrill.

Sartre J-P (1955) *Being and Nothingness*. New York: Philosophical Library.

Silven D and Caldarola TJ (1989) The HIV-positive client. In: Dilley JW, Pies C and Helquist M (eds) *Face to Face: A Guide to AIDS Counselling*. University of California, San Francisco: AIDS Health Project.

Tschudin V (1991) *Counselling Skills for Nurses* (3rd edition). London: Baillière Tindall.

# CHAPTER 6

# Working Together

*Work in a collaborative and co-operative manner with other health care professionals and recognise and respect their particular contributions within the health care team.*

The explosion of knowledge that has occurred this century has made it impossible for one person to possess all the knowledge and skill required to treat the sick in society. This has resulted in new professional groups emerging, many of them, such as physiotherapy and radiography, evolving from tasks at one time included in nursing. While this has enabled highly qualified and skilled practitioners to deal with specific aspects of patient care it has also meant that teams of people have had to come together to ensure that all aspects of care are adequately covered.

## Working in a team

Working in a team is therefore a common experience for today's health professionals and one with which all nurses are familiar. A typical ward team will comprise a ward sister or charge nurse, other qualified nurses (staff nurses), learners, physiotherapists, possibly physiotherapy students, a social worker, perhaps a speech therapist and maybe others. There will also be the medical staff, consultant physicians or surgeons, registrars, house officers and medical students attached to the 'firm'. In addition there may be a ward clerk, a ward receptionist, auxiliaries and domestic workers. A formidable array of people all there ostensibly to 'care for the patient'.

However this apparently common goal may not be perceived as

important in the short term by any of the people mentioned. The medical consultant may be concerned to demonstrate efficiency by achieving a high bed occupancy. The ward domestic may have as her goal the best polished floors in the hospital; the student nurse may want the opportunity to carry out new techniques; the medical student may be concerned with interesting cases, and so on. None of these goals is necessarily bad in itself provided the needs of the patients remain paramount, and this can be achieved by good leadership. But who is the leader of this team? The medical consultant may consider that as it is normally a medical decision to admit or discharge patients, the team leader must be a doctor, yet the ward sister is frequently described as the co-ordinator of care and that may be considered as a leadership role. For a patient whose main aim is to learn to walk again after illness, the physiotherapist may seem to be the key person. Research into the continuity of care of geriatric patients identified the fact that personalised care under the authority of the nurse resulted in a more effective regime than care under the control of the doctor. Experimental National Health nursing homes and units within the Oxford Regional Health Authority have utilised this approach. In these institutions the nurse has the authority both to admit and discharge the patient and to call in medical staff when needed, on a true 'consultancy' basis. In this case the nurse is obviously the team leader.

What is essential is that each individual recognises the contribution that can be made by the others involved in the care of patients so that the most appropriate skills are utilised. Competition is not the most effective way to ensure that the goals relating to patient cure and care are best achieved. As the Code states, the nurse should 'work in a collaborative and co-operative manner with other health care professionals and recognise and respect their particular contribution within the health care team'.

Although this phrase specifies fellow 'professionals' no discussion on team-work in health can ignore the contribution of relatives, voluntary workers and indeed the patient or client as part of the team, as discussed in the previous chapter.

The question may be raised, here, as to whether all team members are of equal worth. The answer raises another question: equal in what sense? Obviously not all have the same knowledge or skill: some will have different attitudes and, as already discussed, individual goals may vary. Nevertheless if all are needed for the effective care of the patient then all should be equally valued for their contribution. The apostle Paul expressed this most succinctly when considering the part played by the members of the church in Corinth. He compares the church to the human body in which each part is different yet all are essential to the full and effective functioning of the person: 'if all were one part, where would the body be?' As it is there are many parts but one body. The eye cannot say to the hand 'I don't need you!' And the head cannot say to the feet, 'I don't need you!' On the contrary, those parts of the body that seem to be weaker are indispensable – so there should be no division in the body, but its parts should have equal concern for each other.

## The medical profession

The doctor has often been accorded supremacy within the team, partly due to the fact that, as already discussed, it is often a medical prerogative to admit and discharge patients. However there are other factors which also tend to ensure that the doctor is seen as more important than the other team members. One important factor is that until recently the doctor has been the only member of the team who has had the benefit of higher education, and hence other team members such as nurses have felt unable to challenge his views on the way in which patients are perceived and/or treated. That situation is changing and one of the comments made about nurses who have taken a degree in nursing is that they are not afraid to question decisions made by the medical members of the team. The fact that traditionally doctors were men and nurses women has also had an effect on the way they perceived each other and that, coupled with the generally higher social class of the doctor over the nurse, has further served to enhance their status. Once again the situation is changing. There are now many women in medicine and an increasing number of men in nursing and these factors may help to change traditional feelings and ensure that people are accorded the respect and status that they earn rather than have their position in the team ascribed to them merely by virtue of the role that they fill.

Occasionally conflict occurs within teams, usually due to the team members holding different goals or values regarding care and cure. Sometimes these values are related to fundamental issues such as the practice of euthanasia, abortion or genetic engineering. In these cases open, honest discussion between all members of the team, including the patient, is essential and where agreement cannot be reached, and the law does not provide guidance, provision must be made for conscientious objection so that any individual team member can withdraw from the situation. In one sense it is important that the individual is seen to be accountable to himself and this requires the person to be able to make decisions regarding actions that enable him to 'live with himself'. The right to make a stand on contentious grounds should be possible without any organisational or professional backlash. To ensure the safety of the patient the individual should ensure that his or her views are known in advance of the specific situation arising so that withdrawal is anticipated.

## Trust hospitals and contracts

The setting up of independent trust hospitals has placed emphasis on 'value for money' and 'contracting' in the provision of services. While no one can quarrel with the desire to achieve efficiency and value for money in the provision of health care there may be occasions when patient need and hospital efficiency clash. The nurse is in a difficult position in that the decisions are made by management and as an employee, the nurse may be bound to abide by them. Some trusts have tried to write into nurses' contracts of employment phrases which bar any criticism of the trust's practices. This may result in conflict as the nurse may see conditions applied which are detrimental to patient care. Once again, this is an area demanding tact and persistence with statements supported by factual material. However, the nurse must not forget that despite managerial loyalty, the patient must not suffer due to silence. The nurse is the patient's advocate.

One of the benefits of team-work is that a new member of the team may receive support from more experienced members who will provide the novice with a variety of role models. Not that learning is restricted to the new member, all team members can and should learn from each other. This is as true for the patient as for the professionals. What is required from all is honesty, trust in each other and a respect for the contribution made by each individual.

## Complaints procedure

Unfortunately, there are occasions when despite repeated approaches to management, accompanied by appropriate evidence, nurses are frustrated in their attempts to change inappropriate practice. What is to be done? It may be necessary to go to the next higher authority and so on. Such activity obviously may cause anger among senior staff and result in individuals or groups of nurses being victimised. In order to help nurses who find themselves in this difficult situation, the Royal College of Nursing has set up a mechanism whereby any nurse can go to receive help, advice and if necessary the backing of the College to ensure not only that patients do not suffer because of their failure to get bad practice changed but also to try to ensure that the nurse or nurses reporting these practices are not victimised by management.

## Questions for reflection and discussion

1. What would you do if you felt that patients' rights were being compromised?
2. What are the benefits and shortcomings of working in a team?

### References

American Hospital Association (1973) *A Patient's Bill of Rights.* New York: AMA.
Apostle Paul 1 Corinthians Chap 12 Verses 19–23. *Holy Bible.* New International Version.

# CHAPTER 7

# Customs, Values and Spiritual Beliefs

*Recognise and respect the uniqueness and dignity of each patient and client and respond to their need for care, irrespective of their ethnic origin, religious beliefs, personal attributes, the nature of their health problems or any other factor.*

We live in a multiracial, multicultural society. Statement six of the Code requires of nurses that they take account of the customs, values and spiritual beliefs of patients or clients.

Customs are a person's regular or established ways of behaving. They are often linked to that person's country of birth, to their upbringing, life experience and belief systems. For some, customs are so ingrained that they are carried out unconsciously, others (and particularly if they are linked to a particular spiritual belief or value system) are very precisely carried out with attention to ritual. Because customs of any sort are embedded so deeply in the background and experience of the person it is important that the nurse respects individual differences, for to question a person's customs is to question that person's self-concept.

A problem arises here as to how nurses can recognise other people's customs. Sometimes the behaviour of other people, if it is unusual, may seem unintelligible or irrational. If this is the case, then it is easy to dismiss a person's customs as peculiar behaviour. What is perhaps essential, is that nurses develop (a) a background knowledge of a variety of examples of customs that relate to particular groups of people and (b) an understanding and clarification of their own customs.

## Customs

In order to develop an understanding of the variety of customs that relate to particular groups of people it is necessary to draw on a number of sources. A shortlist may include: anthropology, geography, sociology, psychology and theology. Anthropology can help in placing people in a particular cultural and social situation (Fox, 1975) and can aid in developing a deep perspective on different styles and ways of living together in a particular country or culture. Geography gives clues as to particular life-styles based on location in the physical world, for example life in a mountainous area or in low temperatures. Sociology offers an analysis and possibly an explanation of how and why people form groups, co-operate, fight and generally exist in a state of interdependence (Chapman, 1977). Psychology offers a closer focus on the individual and suggests a variety of theories about the nature of individual thinking, feeling and behaving. It must be borne in mind, however, that much of the sociological and psychological literature is Western in its orientation. It is an open question as to the degree to which such Western thinking can readily accommodate cultural differences. In other words, can a theorist working and thinking in the West truly understand and account for the behaviour and customs of those living in the East?

The other 'ology', theology, can explain some of the significance of custom from a religious point of view. Again, the temptation to view one's own view of religion as the 'right' one needs to be resisted. This, of course, poses something of a problem. If a particular set of beliefs is held to be 'true', it is naturally difficult to accept that another set of beliefs may also be 'true'! The ability to acknowledge and accept such ambiguity may be a clear sign of open-mindedness and wisdom.

Each of these disciplines offers a different sort of analysis of human action from a different perspective. The skilled nurse would do well to consider these various perspectives as an aid to developing a rich background from which to view a patient's behaviour and customs. For human action never occurs in isolation, it is always embedded in the particular social and psychological context prevalent at the time.

If time is taken to absorb some of the ideas that can be gained from the disciplines outlined above, those ideas can be used to enable the nurse to clarify her own customs. The questions, here, are 'why do I act in the way that I do and how did I come to adopt these patterns of behaviour?' To answer these questions requires some knowledge of the sociological concept of socialisation and of the psychological process known as introjection. Reflection and introspection are also required.

## Reflection

The first stage in the reflective process is becoming conscious of the fact that we act at all. This may seem a ludicrous statement: surely we all know that we act? A moment's reflection, however, will probably reveal that we do not often notice how we act. Much of our action happens spontaneously and without forethought or attention. What is being suggested here is a willing and conscious attention to what is done and why. Heron (1977) has referred to this process as 'conscious use of the self'. Once a person begins consciously to notice what is being done, it is easier to identify the reasons for doing it.

Having begun this process of noticing, it is then possible to compare that action with the theories or explanations offered for human behaviour by anthropologists, sociologists, psychologists and theologians. In this way we can 'personalise' the theories and come to develop theories about personal behaviour, based on rational thought. This reflective and comparative process can lead to an enhanced degree of self-understanding, without which it is impossible to understand the behaviour and customs of others.

## Values

The process of valuing or holding values consists, according to Raths, Harmin and Simon (1966), of three sub-processes: (a) prizing one's own beliefs and behaviours, (b) choosing those beliefs and behaviours and (c) acting on those beliefs. Like customs, values are deeply grounded in cultural heritage, experience and personal belief systems. Also, like customs, they are part of a person's self-concept: those beliefs or behaviours that are held as important (or valuable) make the individual. Values are things that modify behaviour through a process of self-monitoring. Personal value systems allow or disallow certain actions. As with customs, values vary from culture to culture, from group to group and from person to person. It can never be assumed that other people's value systems are similar to one's own. Thus, in nursing, respect for other people's values is vital.

The process of self-reflection and introspection can again help to identify our own values. An aid to this process is a series of exercises in values clarification offered by Simon, Howe and Kirschenbaum (1978). They argue that many people are unaware of their own value systems and therefore have difficulty in knowing how to make decisions about how to act. Through clearly identifying our values we are better equipped to make decisions about how to live our lives. We are also in a better position to appreciate the difference between our value system and that of other people.

It is, of course, one thing to identify and clarify personal values and quite another to appreciate the effect of that value system on other people. Values are reflected in most of the things that are done and particularly in the way things are said. Thus there is a need to develop the ability to pay attention to our verbal behaviour in order that our value system does not offend other people. Consider, for instance, the following situations:

1. The patient who tells you that they have 'no religion' when an initial nursing process assessment is being made.
2. The patient admitted with AIDS, who talks to you about his gay partner.
3. The unmarried adolescent girl who is admitted because of complications during pregnancy.

In each of these situations, what is said to the patient will reflect a particular value system. Notice that it is not possible to escape from the valuing process. For instance, it may be acknowledged in the above cases that the life situation of each person is acceptable. On the other hand, some or all of these life-styles may be unacceptable. Whether 'accepted' or not, a particular value statement is made. In this sense, there is no neutral ground. What is important, however, is that there is acknowledgement that whatever position is held, that of other people is equally valid. A nurse is on difficult ground if condemning others for the values that they hold and on even more difficult ground if that condemnation is verbalised. Such behaviour is not in keeping with the Code of Conduct nor in keeping with the process of caring for others.

## Spiritual beliefs

Linked to the question of values is that of spiritual beliefs. In order for nurses to consider thoughtfully other people's spiritual beliefs it is important that they appreciate the basic differences between various sorts of faiths and, indeed, ways of living without a set of religious beliefs such as atheism, agnosticism and secular human-ism. Spiritual issues have been defined elsewhere as those that are concerned with personal meaning or how we make sense of the world around us (Burnard, 1987). That meaning may be framed in religious terms or it may not. The person who adopts an atheis-tic, agnostic or secular humanistic position is still creating mean-ing, it is just that such meaning does not necessarily include a concept of God. It is worth considering, then, the basic tenets of the major religions of the world and the non-religious philosophies that enable people to create meaning.

**Christianity**

While Christianity can be divided into at least the Orthodox Church, the Protestant Church and the Roman Catholic Church, there are certain tenets of faith that are common to all three. Within each of the main divisions also exists a wide range of different sects and denominations. All major Christian churches believe in the historical significance of Jesus of Nazareth as the son of God, born of a virgin. The essence of Christianity can be identified in the Apostles' Creed:

> I believe in God the Father Almighty, Creator of heaven and earth: and in Jesus Christ his only Son, our Lord who was conceived by the Holy Spirit, born of the Virgin Mary: suffered under Pontius Pilate, was crucified, dead and buried, he descended into hell; the third day he rose again from the dead and ascended into heaven; is seated at the right hand of God the Father Almighty; from thence he shall come to judge the quick and the dead. I believe in the Holy Ghost; the holy Catholic Church; the Communion of Saints; the Forgiveness of sins; the Resurrection of the body, and the life of the world to come. Amen.

The word 'Catholic' in this passage refers to the notion of univer-sality and is not synonymous with the Roman Catholic Church. Christians of all denominations (and a great many of them are described by Sampson, 1982), celebrate the following principal festivals: Christmas, Lent, Good Friday, Easter Sunday and Whit-sun (Pentecost). However, there are a great number of variations of practice in individual denominations and sects. It cannot be assumed that all Christians believe the same things beyond the basic tenets identified above. The theological and doctrinal posi-tion adopted by different denominations varies greatly as does the attention paid to the role of ritual and ceremony. These variations are vitally important to individual believers and are well articulated by Sampson (1982) and Rumbold (1986).

## Judaism

Judaism is a religion essentially of a particular people, the Jews. The history of Judaism and much more of its theological basis can be found in the Old Testament of the *Holy Bible*. The Law of the Jewish people is written in the *Torah*, or first five books of the Old Testament. They await the Messiah and do not recognise Jesus of Nazareth as that Messiah. Important Jewish festivals include: Rosh Hashanah (Jewish New Year), Yom Kippur (the Day of Atonement), Succoth (Feast of Tabernacles), Simchath Torah (Rejoicing in the Law), Chanukah (the Feast of Esther), Purim (the Feast of Lots), Pesach (the Passover) and Tishah B'Av (Mourning for the Destruction of the Temple). Orthodox Jews require their food to be prepared following a specific ritual, and abstain from certain types of meat, notably pork.

## Hinduism

Hinduism is an ancient religion, originally centred in India and Nepal but which has spread wherever Indians have settled. Hindus believe that there are many gods but that all of these are manifestations of one God. Hinduism has no fixed creed and is a very diverse religion. There is a variety of schools of Hindu philosophy and a number of separate religions have developed from it including Buddhism. In the Hindu religion the cow is regarded as a sacred animal and therefore beef is not eaten.

## Islam

The religion of Islam is followed by Muslims. Islam, literally, means submission and Muslims are committed to submitting themselves to the will of God. In the Islamic faith, God is called Allah and Muslims believe Him to be the one true God. They consider Mohammed to be the last great prophet following chronologically after the Jewish prophets and Jesus Christ and they follow his teachings. Again, for Muslims animals used for food need to be prepared in a ritual manner.

Clearly, this cannot claim to be an exhaustive description of the religions under discussion nor does it claim to be a comprehensive listing of all the world's religions. As we have noted, there is already a considerable literature on the topic, to which the reader is referred. It is important in this context, however, to note the considerable variations in the ways in which different cultures give meaning to religious experience. Given the multicultural nature of our society, it is important that all nurses have some appreciation of these varieties of religious interpretation and respect for the differences between them.

Finally, we may consider the issues of atheism and agnosticism. Both are dimensions of spirituality in that both are aspects of some people's belief systems or their attempts to create meaning. Both may be equally respected in the manner that 'religious' beliefs are respected.

## Atheism

Atheism is the unequivocal denial of the possible existence of God. The atheist is the 'unbeliever', the person who does not believe in God. It is interesting to ponder on our individual reaction to such a position. For instance, it is possible to respond by seeing such a person as 'wrong', or that such a person needs only to reflect further for clarification; or that they need more education in order to bring them to the truth. Or can they be accepted as they are? Various reactions are possible; the least acceptable seems to be the notion that somehow the believer is 'right' and the unbeliever is 'wrong'. Belief in God must necessarily involve a 'leap of faith' (Kierkegaard, 1959). There can be no ultimate scientific proof of the existence or non-existence of God. Individuals either believe or do not believe. Neither does the position of unbelief necessarily preclude any sort of moral position. An unbeliever is quite as able to lead a moral life as is a believer. Indeed, Simone de Beauvoir argued that the unbelievers had to lead a 'more moral' life than the believers for, as there was no final arbiter of right and wrong for the unbelievers, they were necessarily thrown back on their own decision-making as a guide to conduct. The believer can be 'forgiven': the unbeliever must forgive herself.

The atheist has to look beyond a concept of God for meaning. That they have to do that does not mean that they do not have spiritual needs. The spiritual needs of the atheist (in terms of a search for meaning) are just as vital as they are for the believer. Some atheists find that sense of meaning in secular humanism. Secular humanism should not be confused with 'humanistic psychology' (Shaffer, 1978). The base argument of secular humanism is best outlined by Blackham (1986). Briefly, the argument is this: people are alone in that there is no God. Because they are alone, they are responsible for themselves. They also have a joint responsibility for all other persons. In acting for themselves, they should act as though they were acting for all mankind. To do less than this is selfishness and not, so Blackham argues, secular humanism. Such a philosophy offers an immediate sense of meaning: the atheist is responsible for herself and for others. As a result, the 'golden rule' applies: 'treat others as we would wish to be treated'. This then, is the basis for morality and for meaning without recourse to belief in God.

### Agnosticism

The agnostic, on the other hand, is in a slightly different position. The agnostic argues that, because it is impossible to prove or disprove the existence of God, silence on the issue is the only wise position (Bullock and Stallybrass, 1977). The agnostic is neither believer nor unbeliever, he holds the view that discussion about the matter is necessarily misplaced, in the end, because such an issue can only ever be a matter of faith. Again, such a position does not, of itself, rule out the need for meaning or morality. The agnostic, like the atheist, still needs to discover or invest life with meaning in what they do or how they live. Some may argue that the only meaning that can be found in life is that which individuals invest it (Kopp, 1972). In other words, there is no ultimate meaning for the way things are: *people* bring meaning to their actions. Meaning, therefore, is an intrinsic concept and dependent upon the individual's reasoning or perception.

These are thumbnail sketches of two positions alternative to that of belief in God. There is, of course, another position, that of the person who either does not know whether or not he believes in God and a further position, that of the person who does not believe such issues to be important. It is argued here that such positions are just as valid as those adopted by people who claim to be believers.

There are many situations in which such positions need to be considered in nursing. As we have seen, one of the questions asked on admission of a patient may relate to that person's 'religion'. Such a question leaves no doubt that the accepted position is that of 'believer'. Indeed, it is quite possible that many patients, in this culture, faced with the question and uncertain about their own beliefs, will answer 'Church of England' or 'Catholic', whether or not they are members of those churches, in order not to embarrass themselves. It may take considerable bravery to answer 'none' or 'atheist' in these circumstances! We need to think long and hard about how we may pose questions of belief or unbelief without making such questions leading questions.

Also, it is necessary to consider the sorts of value-judgments nurses may make about other people's belief systems. If the nurse is a believer, is there a harsh judgment of the unbeliever? If, on the other hand, the nurse is an unbeliever, is the believer dismissed? It is important that there is an acknowledgement that either belief system may not coincide with that of the patient. Nor is it appropriate that nurses proselytise or evangelise for either position. Nurses, in the role of carers, are not required to convert others to belief or unbelief.

There are other, more delicate questions. Acceptance, for instance, of the fact that the unbeliever may not see the need for the conventional funeral service. 'Secular' forms of service are available through national secular societies. It may also need to be acknowledged that death may not be a fearful event for the unbeliever, nor need it be a fearful event for unbelieving relatives.

The whole question of belief and value systems underlies the way nurses approach the issue of patients' spiritual needs. Nurses must first clarify their own belief and value systems before they are clearly able to help patients with such 'ultimate' questions. Values clarification exercises may be useful here (Simon et al., 1978). So may open discussion in schools of nursing of all aspects of spirituality, both religious and secular.

It would do great disservice to a wide variety of ways of addressing spiritual matters if the term 'spiritual' was only connoted as being to do with religious matters. Nurses clearly need to be open-minded in their approach to this vital aspect of nursing care.

Finally, David Cooper (1992) offers this useful list of do's and don'ts regarding the care of patients and clients from various cultures.

---

## Name

*Don't* use Western titles, such as Mr, Miss, Ms, Mrs.
*Don't* ask non-Christians for a Christian name.
*Do* ask for family name or first name.
*Do* avoid repetition in clinical notes. Find out the correct family name first rather than misuse several different names.

## Language

*Don't* assume that all ethnic minority groups speak English.
*Don't* assume that all ethnic minority groups do *not* speak English.
*Do* avoid making assumptions by using accurate assessment procedures.
*Don't* use the family to interpret intimate questions.
*Don't* use a family member to break bad news. He or she may avoid the issue if it is believed to be too stressful for the client.
*Do* use an interpreter who understands medical terminology; this will avoid stress for the interpreter and client and also avoid misinterpretation.
*Do* be aware that only women may ask intimate questions of women in some cultures. This will avoid wrong information being passed, and avoid embarrassment.

## Religion

*Don't* generalise about a client's religion.
*Do* remember that for Buddhists, Christians, Jews, Sikhs, Hindus and Muslims, religion may be an integral part of daily life.
*Do* avoid incorrect assumptions; find out the different beliefs and approaches.
*Do* record clearly and make notes of the client's wish to see or have present a representative from his religion.
*Do* ask the family who you should contact if the client is not able to relay this to you.
*Do* remember that many Eastern religions fast on certain days; pray at certain times; wear religious objects or symbols.
*Don't* mistake religious objects or symbols for jewellery.
*Do* check to see if any nursing interventions will compromise any religious beliefs.
*Do* inform the client and/or family of any nursing interventions before commencing, to check religious beliefs.
*Do* check religious observations with client and family.
*Do* consult with religious advisers or teachers to gain permission and/ or to obtain exemption, to allow procedures to take place. Ensure she explains this to the client.

## Diet

*Don't* give Jews or Muslims pork or pork products.
*Do* make sure that other meat offered to Muslims has been naturally slaughtered by the halal method.
*Do* remember that not all Jewish people eat kosher food (specially prepared to make pure).

*Do* remember that not all Muslims eat halal meat.

*Do* consult the client regarding any diet preferences.

*Do* remember that meal times are family occasions in Eastern culture; matters relating to the family are often discussed here.

*Do* remember that being taken out of a close family environment can be frightening and cause loneliness, which may cause loss of appetite.

*Do* invite the family to bring in food and to join in meal times, if at all possible and practical.

## Personal hygiene

*Do* remember that to Sikhs, Hindus and Muslims washing in still water is considered unclean.

*Do* supply the client with a jug of water and a bowl and/or running tap and empty wash-basin to allow hand, face and body washing.

*Do* make exceptions if the client is dependent.

*Do* remember that Muslims use the right hand for eating and food preparation, and the left hand for cleaning themselves and other procedures. Anyone unable to do this because of injury or other health reasons will need counselling and discussion relating to ways of surmounting this problem (it may be useful to supply a plastic glove).

## Modesty

*Don't* compromise the client's dignity and modesty.

*Do* remember that exposure of the female body to a male will cause distress in certain cultures, especially if the client is in purdah (the duration of menstruation).

*Do* offer separate bays in mixed-bedded wards, or if possible a single room, especially for those in purdah.

*Do* remember that hospital gowns often expose more than they cover, and are therefore unacceptable.

*Do* avoid exposure of arms or legs; for example, in the case of a fractured limb. Add additional covering to protect modesty.

## Skin and hair

*Do* remember that Afro hair may be brittle and dry; add moisturiser or oil to the scalp and comb regularly.

*Do* remember to ask the client what they use for skin moisturiser.

*Do* remember that dark-skinned people are prone to kelid scarring (hyperkeratinisation); invasive treatment will cause excessive pigmented scarring.

*Do* remember to inject or undertake invasive procedures in a site that will avoid disfigurement if possible.

*Don't* assume that children of Asian, African or Southern European descent have bruising if you see marks around the sacrum, buttocks, or hand and wrists; these may be Mongolian blue spots.

*Do* avoid accusations of child abuse by undertaking full and proper assessment and advice.

## Hospital procedures

*Do* give careful thought to procedures and routines before commencing them.

*Do* remember that discussing elimination or other intimate health issues may be culturally offensive.

*Do* approach all patients sensitively, ensure privacy and maintain the individual's right to self-respect.

*Do* remember that some medications and treatments may be taboo for some religious groups.

*Don't* give Jehovah's Witnesses blood transfusions.

*Don't* give Muslims, Jews and vegetarians iron injections derived from pigs.

*Don't* give insulin of porcine origin to Jews or Muslims.

*Do* remember that many emollients contain animal derivatives.

*Do* remember that some medications have an alcohol base which may be forbidden in some cultural groups: the client with a drinking problem may wish to avoid these preparations.

*Do* be aware of all preparations likely to contain potentially taboo or offensive ingredients.

## Visiting

*Do* remember that limiting visiting to two people may cause distress in extended family cultures.

*Do* remember that West Indian, Asian and Middle Eastern families like to visit as a family.

*Do* remember that the 'family' may include children, uncles, aunts, grandchildren, parents and grandparents.

*Do* compromise over visiting, and number visiting per bed.

*Do* remember that open visiting can be more accommodating.

*Do* allow the family to participate in the client's care.

## Myths

*Don't* believe that people from different races have low pain thresholds. This is not true, for example:

Japanese may smile or laugh when in pain, thus avoiding loss of face;
Anglo-Saxons may be sullen and withdrawn, portraying the stiff upper-lip image;
Eastern Europeans, Greeks and Italians express pain vocally and freely.
*Do* remember that every individual has a different level of pain tolerance, regardless of race, culture, country of origin or creed.

### Death and bereavement

*Do* involve client and family in the care.
*Do* remember the Eastern cultures like to take an active part in the care of dying relatives, especially last offices.
*Do* remember that in certain cultures, custom and practice will need to be followed if the client is to proceed along the continuum of life following her earthly death.
*Do* ensure that you are fully conversant with specific cultural requirements for death, bereavement and last offices.
*Don't* deny the family the right to participate in last offices as this will increase the pain already being experienced and may slow down the grieving process.
*Do* negotiate to minimise anxiety and allow some participation, when the family's wishes come into conflict with hospital policies and procedures. This will assist the grieving process.
*Do* compromise – the client and family have only one chance to say their goodbyes.

Reproduced from Wright H and Giddey M (1992) *Mental Health Nursing: From First Principles to Professional Practice.* London: Chapman and Hall, with permission.

## Questions for reflection and discussion

1. Are you clear about your own spiritual values?
2. To what degree have *you* been prepared for looking after people from different cultures?

## References

Blackham HJ (1968) *Humanism.* Harmondsworth: Pelican.
Bullock A and Stallybrass O (eds) (1977) *The Fontana Dictionary of Modern Thought.* London: Fontana.
Burnard P (1986) Picking up the pieces. *Nursing Times* **82**(17): 37–39.

D

Burnard P (1987) Spiritual distress and the nursing response: theoretical considerations and counselling skills. *Journal of Advanced Nursing* **12**: 377–382.

Chapman CR (1977) *Sociology for Nurses*. London: Baillière Tindall.

Cooper DB (1993) Transcultural issues and approaches. In: Wright H and Giddey M (eds) *Mental Health Nursing. From first principles to professional practice*. London: Chapman and Hall.

Fox R (1975) *Encounter with Anthropology*. Harmondsworth: Penguin.

Frankl V (1963) *Man's Search for Meaning*. New York: Washington Square Books.

Heron J (1977) *Behavioural Analysis in Education and Training*. Human Potential Research Project. Guildford: University of Surrey.

Kierkegaard S (1959) *Either/Or*. Vol 1. New York: Doubleday.

Kopp S (1972) *If you meet the Buddha on the road, kill him! A modern pilgrimage through myth, legend, Zen and psychotherapy*. London: Sheldon Press.

Raths L, Harmin M and Simon S (1966) *Values and Teaching*. Columbus, Ohio: Merrill.

Rumbold G (1986) *Ethics in Nursing Practice*. London: Baillière Tindall.

Sampson C (1982) *The Neglected Ethic: Religious and Cultural Factors in the Care of Patients*. Maidenhead, Berkshire: McGraw-Hill.

Shaffer JPB (1978) *Humanistic Psychology*. Englewood Cliffs, New Jersey: Prentice Hall.

Simon S, Howe LW and Kirschenbaum H (1978) *Values Clarification*. Revised edition. New York: A and W Visual Library.

# CHAPTER 8

# Conscientious Objection

*Report to an appropriate person or authority, at the earliest possible time, any conscientious objection which may be relevant to your professional practice.*

One of the fundamental rights of any person in the UK is the right to exclusion from any activity on 'conscientious' grounds. Even in wartime an individual who objects in principle to killing another person may request exemption from military service.

There is an important distinction to be made between an individual who objects to an action because of strongly held and soundly based principles and an objection made in a particular situation because at that time there is a conflict of professional judgment. For example it may be possible for a nurse to consider that in many situations treatment by electro-convulsive therapy is a justified treatment but on one specific occasion to consider that the patient is not physically fit to receive such treatment. In this case any objection to the patient receiving the treatment is made on professional grounds and may or may not be accepted by the medical staff in charge of the case. Quite a different situation would apply if the nurse objected to the treatment on the grounds that it was morally wrong to administer a treatment that interfered with the normal function of the brain. In this case it would be appropriate for that nurse to ask to be relieved from participation in the treatment on conscientious grounds.

Obviously objections based on principle will be known ahead of any specific situation arising and therefore the nurse should make such objections known so that appropriate staffing arrangements can be made and the patient adequately cared for.

The basis for such principles may be religious and/or moral. Such principles have to be decided upon by the individual and cannot be the subject of rules.

## Categorical imperatives

The philosopher Kant (1785) endeavoured to lay down guidance for individuals who faced the difficult situation of having to decide on the rightness or otherwise of a course of action. He called his guidelines 'categorical imperatives' thus giving them more strength than perhaps many would accord them. The first of these imperatives states that a person should:

> Act only on that maxim through which you can at the same time will that it should become an universal law.

It is this type of action that is based on a fundamental principle that forms the grounds for conscientious objection. However it is also expected that a nurse will act in such a way that no harm will befall the patient and therefore it is both morally expected and to a degree required by law that a nurse should make clear any reasons that may exist which indicate to her that a proposed course of treatment will not only be of little benefit but may also be harmful to the patient.

It is this type of action that may result in disagreement between health care professionals and which, in an ideal world, would be resolved by open and frank discussion. However this is not an ideal world and if the treatment ordered is the responsibility of another professional, then the nurse may fail to halt its progress. In such a case it would be wise for the nurse to record the objection made and the grounds for dissent. Such a decision is one for the individual to take and is not one that can be solved by resort to hierarchical power or policy statements, nevertheless the nurse lodging an objection may be required to justify the action taken.

The National Board for Nursing Midwifery and Health Visiting for Scotland issued a Guidance Paper for nurses who objected to a medical treatment. In it they suggested that the following steps might be helpful:

1. The person who issued the instructions should be asked for clarification.
2. The nurse expressing concern should provide factual, rationally defensible evidence for her concern.
3. Clearly documented nursing assessments and records are essential.

All the suggestions in this chapter regarding the nurse being able to account for why she wishes to object on conscientious grounds indicate the need for that nurse to identify and understand her own value and belief system. Clearly, a person cannot account for why they object to something if they have not given sufficient thought to the basis for such an objection. The notion that nurses should become self-aware has been discussed more fully in other parts of this book. In the domain of conscientious objection, that self-awareness becomes a particularly important prerequisite. It is vital that all nurses appreciate what their beliefs and values are, why they hold them, what their limitations are and the areas of likely conflict either with others or with the profession. Without such clarification, many decisions of conscience may be made 'blindly' and without due rational thought. It is important, in a professional context, that objections should not be made on a whim but firmly grounded in systematic argument.

## Verbalising objections

Further, it is important that all nurses who wish to object in this way are able to express their objections clearly and to verbalise them appropriately. Such expression may be enhanced by nurses developing assertion skills (Alberti and Emmons, 1982). Assertiveness enables the person to be clear about what they want to say, develop the courage to say it clearly and, if necessary, be prepared to repeat what they have to say. It is arguable that the nursing profession, as it exists at present, has tended to produce complaint and rather unassertive professionals. The hierarchical structure of the medical profession and the tradition that the nurse is somewhat lower in status than her medical colleagues has tended to reinforce this self-image. As we have seen, the profession is changing and so is its relationship with medicine. Perhaps it is time for nurses to develop assertiveness skills – skills which can easily be taught through the medium of experiential learning. In experiential learning sessions, nurses can clarify what it is they have difficulty in saying to others, they can practise being assertive (through role-play and skills rehearsal) and they can receive feedback from their peers as to their effectiveness. Such sessions, if handled well by the facilitator, can increase individual confidence and also make the process of becoming assertive more effective. Like all skills, assertiveness needs practice. While many schools of nursing are currently incorporating the teaching of assertiveness skills into the curriculum, further training is widely available through extra-mural departments of colleges and universities.

## Peer support

Small groups of nurses may also consider setting up peer support groups in order to learn such skills themselves. Ernst and Goodison (1981) offer a wide range of practical suggestions as to how such a group may be set up, how to keep it going and how to understand and cope with the teething troubles that may arise. Indeed, such a group may serve a triple purpose:

1. To develop assertiveness skills.
2. To clarify beliefs and values in the company of supportive colleagues.
3. To enhance self-awareness.

All of these things will make easier the process of deciding whether or not to object to any aspect of nursing or medicine on conscientious grounds.

## Questions for reflection and discussion

1. Could you ever imagine yourself as a conscientious objector?
2. Would you support another person who wanted to be one?

### References

Alberti RE and Emmons ML (1982) *Your Perfect Right: A Guide to Assertive Living*. 4th edition. San Luis, California: Impact Publishers.
Ernst S and Goodison L (1981) *In Our Own Hands: a Book of Self-help Therapy*. London: The Women's Press.
Kant I (1785) *Fundamental Principles of the Metaphysics of Morals* (trans. Abbott TK). New York: Library of Literal Arts.
National Board for Nursing Midwifery and Health Visiting for Scotland (1985) Guidance Paper: *Questioning of, or Objecting to, Participation in Medical Procedures*. Edinburgh: SNB.

# CHAPTER 9

# Privileged Relationships

*Avoid any abuse of your privileged relationship with patients and clients and of the privileged access allowed to their person, property, residence or workplace.*

The relationship that develops between a patient or client and a health care worker is unique. Unlike the relationships in which individuals normally become involved, this one is usually one in which neither the patient, client nor the nurse has any real choice. Apart from the situation where an individual engages a specific private nurse the patient has no say as to who is selected to provide care. Equally the nurse is rarely able to choose the patients allocated to her care or to opt out of involvement. So the situation is one where two individuals who may have little in common socially or in any other way find themselves in an intimate interaction.

In addition the nurse is likely to have access to information not normally disclosed to other people and may be involved in activities that breach customary social taboos. For example in Western society it is not normal for a male person to be seen naked by a young female, except in a close family relationship. The uniqueness of the situation is often remarked upon by older male patients who say wryly that the nurse is 'young enough to be my daughter'. Alternatively many female patients feel embarrassed if examined or cared for by a male doctor or nurse. However the discomfort is not always experienced by the patient; nurses may also feel uneasy in some situations, finding it difficult to separate normal social expectations from the relationships not only permitted but demanded in intimate patient care.

It is not only in the physical sphere that the relationship may be

95

unusual, a ward will contain a wide range of individuals with different education, employed in a wide range of occupations and belonging to different social classes. There will also be a wide range of individual differences between patients in terms of personality type, personal preferences, values, beliefs and perceptions. However as far as the nurse is concerned these factors must make no difference to the way in which they are treated or receive care.

In a small community it is possible that a patient may already be known by the nurse, either personally or because of the position they hold in the community. It is vital that in this case the nurse is able to detach herself from this personal knowledge to ensure impartiality. Equally any knowledge gained during the professional relationship must not be used outside the professional interaction.

## Community nursing

Community nurses have an additional privilege in that they are able to enter the home of their clients. Once again this will provide knowledge about the home that would not normally be available except to chosen friends. Sometimes the patient's way of life will be such that the nurse may dislike or even disapprove of it. However, unless it has a bearing on the health of the patient, comment should not be made nor should the details be related to other people.

The occupational health nurse has another concern. While her responsibility is the health and/or safety of the worker, management may be anxious to receive information about the worker for organisational reasons. It may be difficult in certain circumstances to separate what information is of a privileged nature and therefore confidential and what can legitimately be used by the management. The decision has to be made on the basis of whether it would have been given in any situation other than to the nurse.

Often when the relationship between the patient and the nurse is prolonged, a friendship over and above that of a professional relationship may develop. It is in this situation that the greatest care has to be taken to avoid abusing the relationship. It is important, here, to consider the power-relationship that exists between nurse and patient. In almost all such relationships, the nurse is necessarily in a dominant position *vis-à-vis* the patient. This is often due to the fact that the patient is always dependent upon the nurse, it is never a case of the nurse being dependent on the patient. Thus, the relationship is unequal.

This unequal relationship may echo the earlier parent–child relationship and may be similar to what, in psychotherapy, is known as 'transference' (Procter, 1978; Schafer, 1983). When transference occurs in the nursing relationship, the patient comes to view the nurse as having all those positive qualities that she once saw in her mother or father. (This is 'positive' transference. In 'negative' transference, the patient sees in the nurse all sorts of negative parental qualities. Fortunately, in nursing, this negative transference is likely to be less common.) This unconscious mental process may lead to the patient becoming very dependent upon the nurse. Examples of this happening may be when the patient suggests that a particular nurse is 'her' nurse or is 'more understanding' than other nurses. Such compliments may be very flattering to the nurse and are, of course, genuinely felt by the patient. All nurses need to be aware that this deeper level of dependence may occur and that it may bring with it the desire in the patient to ask for a closer relationship with that nurse.

## Saying goodbye

It is particularly important for the longer term nurse–patient relationship to be 'ended' gently and slowly by the nurse concerned. The process of 'saying goodbye' should be considered as soon as the nurse realises that an end to the relationship is in sight. Very often the patient who has become very dependent will deny to herself that the end of the relationship is going to occur at all. In this case, the patient continues to act as though the relationship will carry on indefinitely and may be very hurt by the ultimate ending of it. It is easy for the nurse to underestimate how much a nurse–patient relationship can mean to the patient. It is vital, however, that the nurse can differentiate between a professional relationship and a friendship. While it is tempting to think that there need be no differentiation between the two and that patients can be 'friends', such a position fails to acknowledge the complex set of psychological processes that may be occurring when a dependent, often sick, person is meeting a 'care giver'. The relationship that develops out of this set of circumstances is usually very different from the circumstances that surround the more usual development of a friendship. In an ordinary friendship, the two people involved are usually of relatively equal status and are free to choose whether or not they become emotionally attached to each other. In the nurse–patient relationship, as we have seen, the two people involved do not informally 'choose' each other but find themselves together in a complex web of emotional, physical and social circumstances.

## Psychiatric nursing

In psychiatric nursing, the need to appreciate the boundaries of relationships is, perhaps, even more acute. The nature of the psychiatric nurse–patient relationship is such that the patient will often disclose to the nurse a considerable amount of their personal feelings and such disclosure can lead to dependence. It is important that the psychiatric nurse has a strong sense of her 'ego boundary' – of the difference between her own identity and the identity of the patient. Thus, a degree of self-awareness is required here: through understanding something of our own makeup, we learn to discriminate between ourself and the other person (Bond, 1986; Burnard, 1985). Without such awareness there is a danger of blurring the distinction between our personal feelings and the feelings of the patient. Such blurring of roles and identities leads to confusion on the part of the patient and can lead to emotional exhaustion on the part of the nurse.

In the past, nurses were encouraged never to become emotionally involved with patients. In recent years the notion of being able to be totally objective in relationships has been called into question. Perhaps, in the end, it is a question of balance and of being able to judge the issue of 'therapeutic distance'. If, on the one hand, the nurse stands too far back from the patient, she will be unable to empathise. In this case, she stands in what Martin Buber (1958) called an 'I-it' relationship to the patient: the patient is in danger of becoming an 'object', or a 'thing'. A classic example of how patients may be turned into things through this distancing is seen whenever a patient is referred to by diagnosis – 'the appendix in bed six'. If, however, the nurse stands too close, she will be so involved that she will find it difficult to sort out her own emotions from those of the patient. The skill lies in establishing the optimum point in which to stand in relation to the patient – neither too detached, nor too involved: a relationship that Buber called the 'I-thou' relationship and one in which both parties meet as human beings – counsel of perfection, perhaps! In everyday life, such emotional distances are extremely hard to judge but the onus should be on the nurse to endeavour to make such judgment.

# Friendships

Sometimes, of course, friendships between nurses and patients do extend beyond the initial nurse–patient relationship. The point, here, is not that such relationships should never occur, but that the nurse has particular responsibility in considering the power balance in the relationship and should consider very carefully whether or not a friendship that develops out of such a nurse–patient relationship is one freely chosen by the patient. It may seem strange to question whether or not friendships are 'chosen' in this way but it may be even stranger to call a state of dependence a friendship. Just as a psychotherapist would be acting unethically if she took advantage of the strong emotions aroused in her client by the close relationship engendered by psychotherapy, so the nurse should not exploit the often equally strong emotions invoked by the administration of care.

Some situations produce particular problems, as when a patient or client is of particular interest to the Press. It is obvious that journalists have a job to do and equally obvious that they have readers avid for details of the personal lives of celebrities. In order to meet this need for information they often ask what appear to be innocuous questions which may be acutely embarrassing when used out of context. In order to avoid this problem most health authorities have a press officer and it is important that she is the only person who speaks to media representatives.

One of the first things that any nurse needs to learn is that apparently harmless gossip about who is in the ward or who has been into a clinic may be inappropriate and in particular such chat in a public place such as on a bus or train can be overheard and possibly misused.

From this discussion it can be seen that the nurse is in a very privileged position, interacting with a wide variety of people, allowed access to information and buildings and made privy to intimate details relating to individuals and families. This privilege carries with it the responsibility not to abuse this unique position.

## Questions for reflection and discussion

1. In your experience, what have been the most difficult things about 'saying goodbye'?
2. What, for you, would constitute misuse of a privileged relationship?

## References

Bond M (1986) *Stress and Self-Awareness: a Guide for Nurses.* London: Heinemann.

Buber M (1958) *I and Thou.* 2nd edition. New York: Scribner.

Burnard P (1985) *Learning Human Skills: a Guide for Nurses.* London: Heinemann.

Proctor B (1978) *The Counselling Shop.* London: André Deutsch.

Schafer R (1983) *The Analytical Attitude.* New York: Basic Books.

# CHAPTER 10

# Confidentiality

*Protect all confidential information concerning patients and clients obtained in the course of professional practice and make disclosures only with consent, where required by the order of a Court or where you can justify disclosure in the wider public interest.*

Clause 10 of the Code of Professional Conduct emphasises that confidential information obtained in the course of professional practice should not be disclosed without the consent of the patient or one authorised to act on the patient's behalf apart from three exceptions: the requirements of the law, by order of a Court, or in the public's interest.

Such a statement would appear to state self-evident facts, however the issue of confidentiality raises many questions, so many in fact that the UKCC issued an elaboration of clause 10 in an effort to clarify some of the queries raised.

The need for confidentiality is one that was recognised as far back as the compilation of the Hippocratic Oath in which newly qualified doctors are asked to declare:

Whatsoever things I see or hear concerning the life of men, in my attendance on the sick or even apart therefrom, which ought not to be noised abroad, I will keep silence thereon, counting such things as sacred secrets.

As the UKCC's document explains, the focal word in the definition of confidentiality is 'trust' and without this trust no therapeutic relationship can be developed or maintained between the health care worker and the patient or client.

The level of trust placed by the patient in the doctor or nurse is very high indeed. It results in the disclosure of personal details, the submission to intimate examination both physical and mental and the agreement to, and co-operation in, often unpleasant treatment regimens. In return for this trust the patient has the right to expect that information given and details of mind and body revealed will be respected and only used in a therapeutic manner.

## Rights and duties

This is an interesting example of the fact that rights and duties are in effect opposite sides of the same coin. In the doctor– or nurse–patient relationship the pattern is as shown in Table 10.1.

| Doctor/nurse | | Patient/client | |
|---|---|---|---|
| Right | Duty | Right | Duty |
| Information | Confidentiality | Knowledge | Reveal data |
| Access to mental/ physical data | Treatment | Confidentiality | Co-operation |

**Table 10.1**   The pattern of the doctor– and nurse–patient relationship

By agreeing to enter into a relationship with a health care professional the client tacitly agrees to divulge appropriate information to him. However, one of the potential problems relating to the maintenance of confidentiality is that in most cases the person is not cared for by one individual but by a team made up of a wide variety of workers. In this situation it is essential that all the team members have access to the relevant information and generally patients are aware of this fact and therefore their consent to the availability of data is implied.

One problem is to decide who the team members really are and therefore who should have access to records. It may be clearly understood by a patient that the doctor and nurse need information and probably few would question the physiotherapist's right of access to the patient's file, but has the hospital chaplain the same right of access and what should be the position of the wide range of students who may be involved in the organisation?

The patient may regard some personal information of such a sensitive nature that a request is made that access to it be restricted. This request should be honoured and if subsequently it becomes apparent that an individual not originally considered to need the information is found to require it for the good of the patient, then specific permission to share that knowledge must be obtained.

This can cause difficulties in some cases, for instance a patient may confide in a nurse and request that no other person be told, yet the nurse may recognise that this information is needed by the doctor if appropriate action is to be taken. In this case the nurse should not divulge the information but explain to the patient why it is vital for the doctor to be told and the disadvantage that secrecy may cause.

## Accidents

Even more difficult is the situation occurring when a nurse or doctor is told, or finds out by accident, details which may not directly affect the patient's care but have major implications for the rest of society. An example of such information may be evidence of criminal activity such as trafficking in drugs or child abuse.

The Code itself highlights this potential difficulty in that the opening paragraph talks about 'acting at all times in the interests of society' yet emphasises that 'above all the interest of individual patients and clients must be safeguarded'. However clause 9 does allow for disclosure in exceptional cases, 'when the law requires it, when the court orders it or when it is necessary in the public interest'. The UKCC's leaflet in discussing this dilemma recognises the strain this situation may place on the individual practitioner who has to decide when disclosure is not only permissible but also necessary. The recommendation is that the practitioner should seek advice from other practitioners not only nurses, midwives and health visitors, but also other professionals. In addition it may be both wise and helpful to consult with the appropriate professional organisation. The implications of the disclosure of information must be considered from all angles before the final decision is reached.

While the discussion so far has focused on the professional's responsibility to maintain confidentiality, the DHSS Working Group on Confidentiality has suggested that employment contracts of those who handle confidential records, for example medical secretaries and record clerks, should contain the following clause:

> In the course of your duties you may have access to confidential material about patients, members of staff or other health service business. On no account must information relating to identifiable patients be divulged to anyone other than authorised persons, for example medical, nursing or other professional staff, as appropriate, who are concerned directly with the care, diagnosis and/or treatment

of the patient. If you are in any doubt whatsoever as to the authority of a person or body asking for information of this nature you must seek advice from your superior officer. Similarly, no information of a personal or confidential nature concerning individual members of staff should be divulged to anyone without the proper authority having first been given. Failure to observe these rules will be regarded by your employers as serious misconduct which could result in serious disciplinary action being taken against you, including dismissal.

The fact that confidential information is contained in personal records has been a contentious issue for many years. Many patients have been suspicious as to what has been recorded, especially as traditional wisdom and many health agency policies deny the patient the right to see these records. The Data Protection Act (1984) legally protects 'automatically processed information' which in practice normally means computerised records. Under this Act any material kept on a computer record for 40 days or over must be available for inspection. However the Act does not cover data processed manually. Data users, that is individuals who control the contents and use of personal data which is automatically processed, must register the type of data that they hold, how it is obtained and the purpose for which it is required.

## The medical profession

The medical profession has been very disturbed by the requirements of this Act, asserting that access by the patient to medical notes might be harmful, break down the trust between the patient and the doctor or inhibit the keeping of full and frank records. In 1986 the British Medical Association voted to urge the Health Minister to exempt medical records from the Data Protection Act. However, to date, this has not been done.

The fact that some records are recorded manually and others automatically may produce an unacceptable anomaly in the patient's right of access to information and it would appear sensible for the same conditions to apply to all records. However it is important to stress that the right of access is held by the individual patient or client and not by relatives (unless in a guardianship role).

The UKCC's document on confidentiality (1987) summarises the principles on which professional judgment should be based in the following manner:

1. That a patient/client has a right to expect that information

given in confidence will be used only for the purpose for which it was given and will not be released to others without their consent.

2. That practitioners recognise the fundamental right of their patients/clients to have information about them held in secure and private storage.

3. That, where it is deemed appropriate to share information obtained in the course of professional practice with other health or social work practitioners, the practitioner who obtained the information must ensure, as far as it is reasonable, before its release that it is being imparted in strict professional confidence and for a specific purpose.

4. That the responsibility either to disclose or withhold confidential information in the public interest lies with the individual practitioner, that he cannot delegate the decision, and that he cannot be required by a superior to disclose or withhold information against his will.

5. That a practitioner who chooses to breach the basic principle of confidentiality in the belief that it is necessary in the public interest must have considered the matter sufficiently to justify that decision.

6. That deliberate breaches of confidentiality other than with the consent of the patient/client should be exceptional.

## The Data Protection Act

Another aspect of confidentiality is the storage of confidential health care information on computers. Anyone who stores information about other people should be aware of their obligations under the Data Protection Act of 1984. The Act recognises the special importance of personal data and the individual citizen's rights. These are expressed in the requirements of the Act which are as follows:

1. All computer bureaux must be registered; all personal data and intended uses for that data must be registered with the Data Protection Registrar and used solely in accordance with the declared objectives of registration. Data may not be sent abroad unless this is specifically permitted by the terms of registration. Individuals about whom data are held (data subjects) have a right to be informed about its nature and contents.

2. Any person owning a computer used to process personal

data (data user), must do so in accordance with the principles of the Act, namely:

personal data shall be processed fairly and lawfully,

personal data shall be held only for one or more specified and lawful purposes,

personal data held for any purpose must be adequate, relevant and not excessive in relation to that purpose or those purposes,

personal data shall be accurate and, where necessary, kept up-to-date,

personal data held for any purpose or purposes shall not be kept longer than is necessary for that purpose or purposes.

The Act also stipulates that an individual shall be entitled at reasonable intervals and without undue expense or delay 'to be informed by any data user whether he holds any personal data of which that individual is the subject and to have access to any such data held by a data user, and where appropriate, to have such data corrected or erased'.

The Act also stipulates that 'appropriate security measures shall be taken against unauthorised access to, or alteration, disclosure or destruction of, personal data and against accidental loss or destruction of personal data' (Peckitt, 1989).

The Act emphasises that the degree of security expected of a data user is related directly to the nature of the personal data and the degree of harm caused by loss, alteration, disclosure or destruction. Users are specifically liable for the physical security of the data, the security of the software system and the reliability of staff having access to the computer.

There are certain exemptions to the Act. In addition to exemption for the private domestic computer user, there are various governmental exclusions – the police, judiciary, revenue services, public data including the electoral roll, and certain financial services. The following classes of data are specifically excluded from the Act:

1. Pay-rolls.
2. Pensions.
3. Accounts.
4. Statistical and anonymous research data.
5. Social services data.
6. Health data of certain sorts.
7. Records held under professional legal privilege (Peckitt, 1989).

All nurses, midwives and health visitors who handle confidential data have a responsibility to ensure that they are clear about whether or not any data that are kept in personal or professional databases are kept legally and within the terms of the Act. Details of registration under the Act are available from The Data Protection Registrar, Springfield House, Water Lane, Wilmslow, Cheshire, SK9 5AX.

## Questions for reflection and discussion

1. Under what circumstances might you break confidentiality?
2. How do you feel about entering into totally confidential relationships?

### References

UKCC (1984) *Code of Professional Conduct*. 2nd edn. London: UKCC.
UKCC (1987) *Confidentiality*. A UKCC Advisory Paper. London: UKCC.
Data Protection Act (1984). London: HMSO.
DHSS (1985) *Report of the Confidentiality Working Group of the DHSS Steering Group on Health Service Information*. London: DHSS.
Peckitt R (1989) *Computers in General Practice*. Wilmslow: Sigma.

# CHAPTER 11

# Caring for Others

*Report to an appropriate person or authority, having regard to the physical, psychological and social effects on patients and clients, any circumstances in the environment which could jeopardise standards of practice.*

The eleventh statement of the Code of Conduct contains a considerable number of important points, some of which have been alluded to in other chapters. It is worth considering each of them in turn.

## The environment of care

First is the notion of the environment of care. What may be said to make up such an environment? One factor which may decide this is where the caring takes place. In a simple sense, the likelihood is that it will either take place in a hospital ward or department or in the patient's home. If the environment of care is a clinical department of a hospital, that environment will contain not only the fixtures and fittings of the ward but also the whole 'climate' of the hospital – the attitudes of the staff, the interpersonal skills demonstrated by such staff and a whole range of almost subliminal things that bombard the patient as a consumer of care. Clearly, then, the nurse has some responsibility to consider her part in creating an environment of care which is, indeed, caring. Care does not stop at offering a range of clinical procedures but includes the whole atmosphere that surrounds the patient during his stay.

In a similar but different sense, the environment of care when it is the patient's home, will also affect that patient's health. While the surroundings may be familiar to the patient, it is likely that they will be perceived in a different way when that person becomes a patient in their own home. Once a person is designated as 'ill' by another family member, that person tends to be viewed differently by the rest of the family and thus will come to view their home circumstances differently. In this sense, then, the 'environment of care' includes the family itself. Again, the nurse needs to take this fact into account when caring for the patient at home.

This leads to the second set of concepts contained in this statement within the Code of Conduct. It asks that the nurse consider the physical, psychological and social effects of the environment on the patient. Most nurses will be familiar with the sorts of physical considerations that must be borne in mind regarding how the environment affects the patient. A shortlist of such considerations would include issues such as heating, lighting, ventilation, freedom from pain, adequate diet, sleep and attention to body functions. There are, of course, many other considerations and the reader is referred to Hunt and Sendell (1983), Du Gas (1983) or Faulkner (1985) for a more detailed discussion of the physical considerations of patient care. In a sense, the main ethical consideration here, is that physical care is carried out thoroughly and with due attention. In some hospitals, this will be further clarified by recourse to a procedure manual of some kind. In others it will be through discussion of a range of principles of physical care.

## Psychological care

The psychological effects of the climate of care are more nebulous and less easy to spell out. We all view the world from a different perspective. How each of us views the experience of illness will vary from person to person. The danger must always be in our generalising about a person's psychological make-up or their psychological reaction to their environment. George Kelly (1955), the personal construct psychologist, noted that if you want to know how someone feels, ask them, they might just tell you! This may give us a useful clue as to how to assess a person's experience of what is happening to them – we ask them and continue to check with them how they are thinking and feeling. This would seem to be a far more appropriate method than assuming how a person is experiencing the world.

This approach may also give us clues as to how to use psychological research and research generated within the field of nursing. It can never be the case that research findings apply to all people in similar situations to those studied in a particular research project. All that research can do is offer us a series of pointers as to what may be the case. Thus we must use research widely and test out whether or not it applies to this person in this set of circumstances. It may or may not.

The same limitation must also apply to the social effects of the caring environment on the patient. For some people, ill health is merely a brief hiccup in their life experience. For others, any bout of illness is something of major concern. Our task as nurses is not to cast value-judgments on how the patient and his family deal with illness but to note how they do, and act accordingly. This again refers back to the notion of sustained awareness, which has been alluded to in other chapters in this book. It is only by constantly observing what patients are telling us that we can make decisions about how to help them. It is notable, too, that all sorts of cultural considerations will prevail, here. People from different countries and cultures view and experience illness in different ways. Nurses would do well to note these cultural differences and, again, not assume that all people experience illness in the same way.

## Caring

What exactly does it mean to care? In the past few years, the concept of care has been widely discussed as an important nursing concept. Milton Mayeroff (1971), in an important analysis of the meaning of caring in human relationships, describes caring as a process which offers people (both carer and the cared for individual) opportunities for personal growth.

Major aspects of caring in the analysis include: knowledge, alternating rhythms (learning from experience), patience, honesty, trust, humility, hope and courage. Those elements are discussed in more detail here although the discussion is a little different from the one that Mayeroff offers.

### Knowledge

To care for someone, we must know certain things. First, we must know who they are. Friendships, for example, develop because as we learn more about the other person, we acknowledge that we like what we get to know. If we did not like it, the friendship would not develop at all. In the context of nursing, we must also get to know the patient in order to get to care for them.

In another sense, however, we need knowledge to *use* and to give to the patient. In the sense of knowledge to use, we need to know certain things about what is wrong with the other person in order to help her. Thus, in caring for a person with heart disease, we need to know various things about the nature of the condition.

It is worth noting, however, that there are definite limits to what we need know in order to care for others. We cannot know very much about what is best for the other person when it comes to their personal or emotional life. It is tempting, when someone has personal problems, to offer them advice. Such advice is only rarely helpful. One moment's reflection will reveal the fact that each of us lives a very different personal life to the next person. While as nurses we can come to know something about the nature of diabetes, we cannot come to know very much about the personal life of the patient. When it comes to personal and emotional issues, the patient is the expert on his own situation. Caring, here, consists of resisting the temptation to tell the patient how to live his life or how to sort out his emotional problems.

**Alternating rhythms**

Any relationship that you have with another person, whether in the family, with friends or with colleagues, does not stay the same. In all these different situations, the intensity of the relationship fluctuates. Sometimes we feel very close to the other person, sometimes we feel quite distant. According to Mayeroff, this is an example of the 'alternating rhythms' of any caring relationship. No relationship (and that includes one with a patient) can stay intense and close for any length of time. There seems to be a natural cycle in the caring relationship – what may be described as the waxing and waning of it.

There is another sense of the term 'alternating rhythms'. This is the idea that we may have to modify continuously the ways in which we react with another person. Sometimes, one approach works. On another occasion, another is required. People vary from day to day. What works with them one day does not necessarily work with them another.

If this is the case, then each new meeting with a person involves us *reknowing* them, with meeting them afresh. Thus, in the context of caring, we must learn this process of remeeting and reknowing the person for whom we care.


## Patience

Caring for another person involves taking your time. While we may hope that a relationship could 'warm up' quickly, very often other people take time to get to know us and to 'allow' the other person to care for them. Again, think of a close emotional relationship that you have with a friend. That relationship did not come about overnight. It took time for both of you to get to know each other and get to like each other. In this sense, then, the caring relationship requires patience. Caring relationships, whether with friends or with patients, cannot be rushed.

In another sense, too, patience requires tolerance. We need to appreciate that other people are not the same as us. We are required, therefore, to accept the person for whom we are caring, 'warts and all'. We cannot hope that the other person will come to be like us. Such a position requires patience: both with the other person and with ourselves.


## Honesty

Honesty is not simply a question of *not* doing things like telling lies or deceiving the other person but involves being open to sharing with them exactly how we feel. It involves being able to tell them the truth, whether that truth consists of factual information that they need, or whether it is concerned with our feelings for them. A prerequisite for being able to be honest with other people is being able to be honest with ourselves. A necessary requirement for being honest with others, then, is a degree of self-awareness, of being able honestly to appraise our own thoughts, feelings, beliefs and values. Put simply, if we do not know certain things about ourselves, we do not know that we do not know them!


## Trust

Just as a child has to be allowed to find things out for himself and to make mistakes so adults must be trusted to learn from their own experience, to make decisions for themselves and so forth. It is easy for nurses to become 'compulsive carers', to smother the person for whom they are caring because they cannot trust that person to take care of himself. Trust, then, also involves 'letting go'. It involves an element of risk taking and accepting that other people find things out in their own way and live their lives differently to us. Often, mistrust in other people demonstrates a distrust of ourselves. In the context of nursing, trust in the relationship is essential. We trust others more when we are secure in ourselves. Thus, again, the need for self-awareness and self-exploration.

## Humility

If another person trusts themselves to us, we need to be aware of the great responsibility that this involves. We cannot afford to become too flattered by the other person turning to us for care. We need to stay humble and to appreciate our own inadequacies and limitations.

If we are not humble, we are likely to feel an overvalued sense of our own knowledge and views. To be humble, however, suggests that we have much more to learn. In the caring relationship, if we stay humble we stay open to new learning and to finding out more about the other person.

## Hope

To care for another person is to affirm that we believe in their ability to overcome problems and adversity. We cannot care without hope. If we do, we may just as well abandon the whole enterprise, for why are we bothering to care at all?

To nurse at all, suggests hope. As we grow fond of someone (which is often, though not always, the outcome of caring) we want to know them more and expect to see more of them. If we do not have hope, then we cannot expect this desire to be fulfilled. In the end, we would not enter into a nursing relationship if we really thought that we had no hope, either for ourselves or for the person whom we were nursing.

## Courage

Despite our efforts, despite our hope, they may *not* recover or, less dramatically, they may not care for us. They may not even like us! Therefore to care is something of a gamble. Just as we cannot know the future, we cannot anticipate the outcome of our caring. Thus to care takes considerable courage.

It takes courage, too, to share ourselves with another person. While caring may not always be a reciprocal relationship, it is likely that we will need to give of ourselves in the caring role. We may also need to tell the person for whom we are caring things about ourselves. As you tell me about you, the unwritten rule is that I tell you about me. In this sense, caring is a process of 'coming to know' the other person. This sharing of self takes courage. We are all vulnerable and all fear that our self-disclosure may not be accepted by the other person. Usually, of course, it is.

These are some of the elements involved in caring for another person. It is not an exhaustive account and often a rather abstract one. Also, it is quite possible to add to Mayeroff's list of aspects of caring in such a way as to highlight a certain arbitrariness in his selection. Suffice to say, though, that unless we care for the client, we are unlikely to be very successful in our counselling.

## Caring attitude

Morrison (1992) has described what he calls the caring attitude: an attitude made up of a variety of themes which attempt to capture the essence of caring in a professional context. The themes that contribute to Morrison's idea of a caring attitude are:

1. Personal qualities.
2. Clinical work style.
3. Interpersonal approach.
4. Concern for others.
5. Level of motivation.
6. Use of time.

These themes seem to move away from the abstract discussion of what it means to care for another person in a therapeutic relationship and begin to offer practical and behavioural indicators of what makes up a caring relationship with another person – particularly in the context of nursing. It is only recently that the whole notion of caring has begun to be researched in a professional context (Watson, 1985; Leininger, 1988). Many of the important issues have yet to be addressed, such as:

1. The inherent contradiction of having 'professional carers'.
2. The question of power and control in the counselling and caring relationship.

3. The 'lived experience' of caring and being cared for.
4. Varieties of caring in different clinical and social settings.
5. The similarities between formal and informal care.
6. The political relationship between the organisation and the individual carer.

## Resources

The next issue dealt with in this section is the reference to having regard to the adequacy of resources. There are in fact at least two issues, here. One is whether or not the patient is receiving the care that he needs. The second, is whether or not resources are available to ensure adequate care. In order to cope with both sides of the equation it is necessary to have a firm sense of both sides: what is available and what is not available. It is no use having plans for a particular style of nursing care if the resources are not available to deliver it. On the other hand it is a pity if we do not deliver the care that we could, because we are not aware of certain resources. In the end, this may be a question of knowledge. We have a duty to make ourselves conversant with the facilities, agencies and policies of the health care environment in which we work.

Linked with this concept of resources is the issue of making known to appropriate persons or authorities any circumstances which could place patients in jeopardy or which militate against safe standards of practice – the final aspect of this statement in the Code. There are a number of issues involved in this notion. First, we must be clear who the 'appropriate persons or authorities' are. Usually, these are spelt out in a grievance procedure or can be obtained from senior nurses or administrators. Second, we need to know the sorts of circumstances which may place patients in jeopardy or militate against safe standards of practice. Again, here a certain level of knowledge is required. We cannot observe unsafe circumstances if we do not have the 'equipment' for making such observations. In this sense, the 'equipment' required is a fund of knowledge from which to draw conclusions. The very least we must have is a sense of our own limitations – of knowing when to ask for an opinion or advice from a more senior colleague. Making decisions about levels of safety are spelt out in a document issued by a particular health authority under the Health and Safety at Work Act, 1974. In other cases such levels are passed on through 'custom and practice'. In either case, it is necessary for the nurse to make an informed decision based on nursing and medical knowledge, appreciation of the facts of the situation at the time and on awareness of current health and safety standards.

## Political awareness

A certain political awareness is also required. We need to be able to formulate questions about why certain standards of conduct and safety exist and how they came to exist. The temptation is to believe that all such standards arise out of rational decisions based on current research and theory! In an ideal world, this would probably be the case but in reality, such decisions are made on much more shaky foundations, including political expedience, tradition, changing ideologies of health care, consumer expectation and even on the basis of crisis management! On many occasions, decisions about standards are made after an incident has occurred – what may be termed retrospectively policy provision. Some of the political issues involved, here, are dealt with by Salvage (1985) and Clay (1987).

## Questions for reflection and discussion

1. In your experience, who are the most difficult people to care for?
2. Do you feel cared for, yourself?

## References

Clay T (1987) *Nurses, Power and Politics*. London: Heinemann.
Du Gas BW (1983) *Introduction to Patient Care: A Comprehensive Approach to Nursing*. 4th edition. Philadelphia: WB Saunders.
Faulkner A (1985) *Nursing: a Creative Approach*. London: Baillière Tindall.
Hunt P and Sendell B (1983) *Nursing the Adult with a Specific Physiological Disturbance*. Basingstoke: Macmillan.
Kelly G (1955) *The Psychology of Personal Constructs*: Vols 1 and 2. New York: Merton.
Leininger MM (1988) History, issues and trends in the discovery and uses of care in nursing. In: Leininger MM (ed) *Care: Discovery and uses in clinical and community nursing*. Detroit: Wayne University Press.
Mayeroff M (1972) *On Caring*. New York: Harper and Row.
Morrison P (1992) *Professional Caring in Practice*. Aldershot: Avebury.
Salvage J (1985) *The Politics of Nursing*. London: Heinemann.
Watson J (1985) *Nursing: Human Science and Human Care: a theory of nursing*. New York: Appleton-Century-Crofts.

# CHAPTER 12

# Reporting

*Report to an appropriate person or authority any circumstance in which safe and appropriate care for patients and clients cannot be provided.*

Item 12 asks that the nurse, midwife or health visitor be able to report, clearly and accurately, any set of circumstances that may endanger the patient. Such an injunction requires a number of skills on the part of the health care professional and these may be identified as:

1. Observational skills.
2. Writing skills.
3. Verbal reporting skills.

## Observational skills

As we have seen at other points in this book, it is essential that all nurses develop their observational skills. A simple experiment will indicate how easily our attention fails us. Put down this book for a moment and become aware of the things that you can see and hear. Allow yourself to notice *everything*: do not attempt to filter anything out. What you will probably discover is that there are many more sounds and many more sights around you that you have wilfully or unconsciously filtered out. This selective filtering process is often essential: if we did not use it, we would become overwhelmed by the inputs of our senses.

On the other hand, we can also *develop* our senses and *choose* to notice what goes on around us. Often, our senses are under voluntary control. Through practice and concentration we can learn to notice much more of what happens around us. It is quite possible to make a contract with yourself to pay close attention to what goes on around you while you are at work. What you notice after work is less important!

Clearly, the more accurate you are in your observation, the more able you will be to report on what you see, if you are called upon to make a written or verbal report.

## Writing skills

If you are required to make a written report, here are some general guidelines that can help.

1. Report only what you *see* not what you *think* you see.
2. Keep to the bare facts. You do not need to include what you think are the rights and wrongs of any given situation.
3. Write short sentences and short paragraphs. Avoid jargon wherever possible and avoid abbreviations that may not be understood by the reader.

Above all, learn to write clearly and simply and do not attempt to use professional jargon just to impress. The aim in professional writing is always to convey information from one person to another. Simplicity in writing is most likely to achieve that aim (Burnard, 1992).

## Verbal reporting skills

You may, occasionally, be called upon to offer a verbal report of an incident. This may be a fairly informal affair – you may, for example, be asked to explain something – or it may be formal – for instance you may be asked to give evidence. Again, the following guidelines may be useful.

1. If you are anxious, be careful not to 'overtalk'. Anxiety can make some people say more than they need or want to.
2. Describe only what you saw or what you did. Do not go beyond what you know to be true.
3. Allow yourself time to think before you respond to a question.
4. Do not be afraid to say that you 'don't know', if this is the case.
5. Keep your replies simple and straightforward and avoid jargon.

# When should you report?

The above paragraphs offer you guidelines on *how* to report, both in writing and verbally. A more difficult question is *when* should you report? The item of the Code suggests that you should be prepared to report 'any circumstance in which safe and appropriate care for patients and clients cannot be provided'. It may be important to identify situations in which this may be the case. Examples might include the following:

1. Staff shortages which mean that certain nursing practices cannot take place.
2. Dangerous or faulty equipment.
3. Situations in which a member of staff is ill or unable to carry out his or her normal duties.
4. Mistakes in prescribing or orders issued by medical or senior nursing staff.

You may wish to consider how this list can be extended. The list divides into those circumstances in which *objects* or *equipment* are faulty and circumstances in which *people* are involved. Clearly, the latter situations are the most difficult ones to make decisions about. At what point, for example, might you report that a member of staff is unable to carry out his or her duties? In the case of a member of staff who was obviously drunk, then the answer might be 'as soon as he came on duty'. If the person is ill however, the situation becomes more complicated. Do you acknowledge the fact at the beginning of a shift and take action then, or do you 'see what happens' and allow some time to elapse before you take action?

When there has clearly been a mistake in prescribing, either drugs or nursing orders, then another set of questions arise. At one level, a mistake can be brought to the attention of the person who made it. This means that all nurses and medical staff must be vigilant regarding each other's actions. A mistake reported to the person who made it may be simply put right. On the other hand, occasions arise in which the person who made the mistake denies that a mistake has been made at all. In this case, it is important that a more senior nurse arbitrates and makes a decision about what should happen next. What happens next may be:

1. An agreement is reached that no mistake has been made.
2. A mistake has occurred and the person who made the mistake should correct it.
3. The 'mistake' should not be translated into action.

E

4. A higher authority should be called to settle any dispute arising from the incident.

In most cases, a written report will have to be made about the incident. It is here that the clear reporting guidelines, identified above, can be used.

## Questions for reflection and discussion

1. How do you rate your own observational skills?
2. Would you say that you write well? If not, what do you need to do to improve your writing skills?

## Reference

Burnard P (1992) *Writing for Health Professionals: a Manual for Writers.* London: Chapman and Hall.

# CHAPTER 13

# Caring for Colleagues

*Report to an appropriate person or authority where it appears that the health or safety of colleagues is at risk, as such circumstances may compromise standards of practice and care.*

In Chapter 5 the role of the various members of the health care team was discussed and their relationship as team members. In this chapter a somewhat different aspect of working together is considered, that of mutual responsibility for each other. It is tempting when all team members have their own areas of responsibility to let each one get on with his own task and assume that each is capable not only of the type of work that they are assigned but that all can work at the same speed and withstand the same pressures. This is obviously not necessarily so.

It is perhaps ironic that while nurses are expected to regard patients as unique human beings entitled to individualised care, they themselves are often regarded as a grade or type and treated as a group rather than as individuals.

This situation exists in all areas of work, in the ward area nurses are often described as 'second years' or 'learners' as if such a title explained everything about that individual; their level of skill, learning needs and so on. The implication is that there is somewhere a template against which each nurse is placed so that each one is identical.

In nursing education a similar situation exists: teaching programmes are formulated in such a way that each learner is expected to learn at the same pace. Rarely is account taken of the fact that individuals start at different levels of knowledge, maturity and life experience. Instead each must conform to a set pattern of teaching methods and, clinical experience, produce almost identical pieces of work for assessment purposes and in every way behave in a predetermined manner. The result is more like the output of a factory rather than the development of an educated professional, able to respond to whatever needs the patient and/or the service may require.

## Sameness

No doubt because of this expectation of 'sameness' that is created by the training programme the same expectation extends throughout the service. Each grade has an area of built-in expectations and standards and anyone who does not fit into the mould is considered to be either slacking, incompetent, a troublemaker or all three.

A moment's thought will demonstrate how unreasonable such an approach is. Physically and psychologically each individual has strengths and weaknesses and therefore, even if two nurses have undergone identical training programmes, it is highly unlikely that they will respond to work pressures in the same way. Link with that their different life experiences, both past and present, their different aims in the profession and in life generally and it will be seen that it is more than probable that each will view their apparent workload differently and react in an idiosyncratic manner to each situation.

Since the advent of a systematic and individualised approach to patient care it is surprising that members of health care teams have not begun to realise that as team members they also are entitled to and should give each other individual care and consideration.

Naturally such an approach is not easy. It is always tempting to feel that if I can cope so should they. Item 11 of the Code states that each nurse should 'have regard to the workload of and the pressures on professional colleagues and subordinates and take appropriate action if these are seen to be such as to constitute abuse of the individual practitioner and/or to jeopardise safe standards of practice'.

# Death

There are many examples of situations where care following death may be needed. One common case is the distress that may occur on the death of a patient. The old, conventional nursing wisdom states that professionals do not allow themselves to become involved with patients and therefore should not be upset when a patient dies. Despite this traditional expectation nurses have always felt grief at the death of a patient and in situations where the patient is seen as an individual not just as a diagnostic category some grief is inevitable and should not be denied. Distress will however vary with the individual nurse and it is important that support is provided by others in the team to those most in need. This may be simple, the provision of a cup of coffee, or more sophisticated as in the provision of counselling or a formalised support group. It is not only nurses who require this understanding and support, the doctor may be equally distressed as may the ward maid, yet these people are rarely considered to need help.

A special example of the need for this type of care may occur when nurses are involved in caring for the victims of a major disaster. Fawcett (1987), the sister in the accident and emergency unit that received the victims of the mass shooting in Hungerford in 1987, describes vividly the fact that during the emergency all the staff worked at a high rate and appeared to be able to cope with the demands being placed upon them. However after the event many demonstrated both psychological and physical disturbance, to quote Fawcett: 'I found my normal emotional resilience had disappeared, and this was made worse by the constant replaying of events in my mind, coupled with insomnia'. In this case support was provided by trained counsellors.

Levels of work may be such as to constitute an impossible load on staff. Nurses are renowned for 'coping' and often see it as a demonstration of failure not to be able to 'get through the work'. Such a situation is often dangerous to those being cared for as in order to fulfil the demands of the workload shortcuts are taken and as a result mistakes made. In addition individuals are often called upon to function at a level for which they have not been prepared and therefore may not be aware of what is safe practice. The misuse and abuse of the enrolled nurse who is frequently required to function as a first level nurse is an example of this latter point. This is an area where nurse managers at all levels have a responsibility to ensure that if adequate levels of staffing cannot be provided, then the clinical area should be reduced or closed. It is very sad to be present at a professional conduct committee and to hear of a nurse who, despite the fact that representation had been made to management, had been left to cope in an impossible situation with the result that a mistake occurred resulting in damage to and sometimes death of a patient.

## Management

It is worth considering, at this point, the manner in which the whole issue of overwork is broached by the person who experiences it, to the manager. Certain social skills are required in order to approach a manager over such an issue and considerable forethought needs to have gone into the presentation. What is required is not that the nurse makes an emotional and, perhaps angry, appeal to the manager but that she prepares a rational and well-thought-out set of arguments as to why she considers she is putting herself or her patients in jeopardy. It is often useful, too, if some possible solutions are identified for discussion with the manager concerned. Very few people like problems thrust upon them either without prior notice or without some ideas for solutions!

Coping with a very heavy workload can be difficult in any circumstances, whether clinical, educational or management. Gortner (1977) offers some principles by which nurses may learn to cope in organisations and manage a heavy and stressful workload:

1. Become competent in what you do. The person who develops the necessary skills and knowledge to do work effectively and efficiently may experience subjectively less stress than the person who does not.
2. Know well the organisation in which you work. It is particularly valuable to become very familiar with the aims of the organisation, the power structure, the hierarchy and the lines of communication. Knowledge of these things allows the nurse to use them effectively to her own and others' advantage.
3. Be a master of the possible. It is useful to identify ways in which aspects of work and/or the organisation can be changed by the individual nurse. Realistic aims that can be reached are usually far less frustrating than highly idealistic ones which may lead to frustration!
4. Recognise and seize the opportunity for doing more. On the face of it, this may seem a curious suggestion for someone who is already working very hard. On reflection, however, it may be identified that it is only through attempting new

projects and developing innovative strategic plans that the individual can develop and 'grow'. There is often a great temptation for the individual to carry on doing those things which she is good at. It is also the route towards boredom and stasis.

5. Consider few problems to be original. Hence the solution is somewhere and that is the challenge. When faced with continuous work pressure, the temptation is to assume that 'nothing can be done' or that 'this situation is so difficult it can never be remedied'. As Gortner (1977) points out, however, few problems are really that new or that difficult. The act of treating them as a challenge can help in the generation of innovative solutions.

6. Recognise the value of support systems. Build and use some for yourself. As we are suggesting in this chapter, colleagues and peers can often be a fruitful source of support. It is often useful if such peer support is formalised and regular peer support groups are set up in which a forum is offered for the discussion of current work-related problems.

7. Know yourself well. A frequent theme running through this book is that of developing self-awareness. One of the first stages in dealing with organisational or work-related stress is knowing personal limitations and areas of vulnerability. This is, indeed, a key practical and ethical issue, for as Shakespeare said 'This above all: to thine own self be true, and it must follow, as the night the day, Thou cans't not then be false to any man . . .' (*Hamlet*, Act 1, Scene 3).

## Burnout

One of the results of continuous work overload may be burnout (Shubin, 1978; Storlie, 1979). This may be defined as an evolutionary and insidious process of growing emotional exhaustion occurring as a consequence of being exposed to chronic job-related stress factors. Three degrees of burnout may be identified. Characteristics of first degree burnout include short-lived bouts of irritability, fatigue and worry and a tendency perpetually to view work situations and colleague relationships in a pessimistic and negative light. Second degree burnout may be viewed as a worsening of the situation, accompanied by feelings of failure, lack of interest in work and a sense of powerlessness and inadequacy. With the onset of third degree burnout comes the development of psychosomatic ailments. Excessive sick leave, the over-use of alcohol and perhaps the excessive use of minor tranquillisers are also symptomatic. With all these changes comes a deep sense of job dissatisfaction. This is often manifest in a sarcastic and cynical manner and a tendency to be judgmental and overcritical of others. A variety of factors may account for the state of burnout. Age and the health status of the nurse are important physical factors. Social factors such as the personal relationships of the individual and the quality of the homelife of that person need to be considered. Environmental factors such as work space, colour, brightness, noise and proximity of other colleagues all play their part. Psychological factors such as the personality of the individual and her problem-solving skills influence the degree to which nurses avoid or develop burnout. Ideological factors such as how authentic the individual feels in her role, the degree to which she feels fulfilled by her job and how much she feels able to invest in relationships with patients all contribute to coping or burning out. Organisational factors such as career position and the rate of organisational change all need to be taken into account.

Because of the insidious nature of burnout or job-related stress, the individual who suffers from it may be unaware that it is happening at all. It falls upon colleagues, then, to be vigilant for signs of it in their colleagues when work pressure is particularly high. While self-monitoring of stress levels is the ideal, it is often impossible for the hard-working person to notice the stress that they are suffering but only too noticeable to those around her! Altruism should not be reserved only for patients but should be freely applied to colleagues. Nursing is, after all, a caring profession.

Charles Kingsley (1885) in his book *The Water Babies* has a character Mrs Do-As-You-Would-Be-Done-By and this could well have served as a heading to this chapter. It may be at some personal cost that a colleague is supported during a period of stress, however it is unlikely that such altruism will go unrewarded as care for each other becomes the norm. The philosopher Kant (1797) expressed the situation in his fundamental principles of morals when trying to lay down rules of moral behaviour which he described as categorical imperatives as follows: 'Act only on that maxim through which you can at the same time will that it should become a universal law'.

Another aspect of this caring for others is the responsibility each person has when delegating work to another to ensure that the person to whom the task is assigned both understands what is required and is capable of carrying it out. This is particularly important when dealing with learners but applies to all aspects of delegation. This is not a one-way responsibility, the person to whom the task is delegated also has the duty to inform the person delegating if the task is not understood or outside her area of competence. Once again this is an area where tradition makes it difficult for some people to admit that they 'don't know how', and it is important that the unit environment is such that individuals do not feel threatened by an admission of ignorance.

Pyne (1987), writing about the formulation of the Code, says:

> Many practitioners now understand that it is respectable to challenge and complain where that is necessary and to accept that to do so is an intrinsic part of proper professional behaviour. I believe that we are steadily observing a revolution in conduct as practising members of the profession accept that the previously held view of 'good conduct' as being compliant and submissive was not only wrong, but responsible for many of the problems that nursing has faced.

While agreeing with these statements it may be necessary in some cases for a nurse to speak up for a less articulate or less confident colleague to ensure that neither the individual is abused nor patients suffer.

## Caring for each other

Implicit in this clause of the Code is the notion of caring for colleagues. Caring is explored in more detail in Chapter 11 but another elaboration of the idea of care may be useful here. In a theological analysis of professional care Campbell (1984) described caring as a form of 'moderated love'. This notion suggested that professional caring relationships were carefully bounded (or moderated) both by custom and by statute. The term 'skilled companionship' (Campbell, 1984) was preferred to that of 'carer' as a description of the relationship that exists between the paid health professional and his patient. According to Campbell, companionship may be differentiated by the following characteristics.

### Closeness without sexual stereotyping

Unlike caring, the idea of companionship is usually devoid of a sexual connotation. Companionship can help to get around the perception of sexual stereotyping such as those commonly found in the health care context: caring as women's work or the suspicion with which men in nursing are typically viewed. Also, and perhaps more contentiously, the idea of romantic love is less likely to be an issue in companionship as it may be in caring.

## Movement and change

Because the idea of companionship is less intense than a full caring relationship, it is more open to movement and change. The carer and the one being cared for are less dependent on each other than is the case in a caring relationship so both can develop and grow at his or her own rate. The other point about movement is that the companion is the person who 'travels with' the other person, who assists, encourages and supports the other to recovery or death. The concept of movement is totally absent in those forms of institutional care where the prevailing norms are stasis, unchanging routine, resigned acceptance and lack of hope. In these circumstances the concept of companionship is lost.

## Mutuality

Companionship suggests mutuality. In accompanying another person we share the relationship and each supports and helps the other. The *degree* to which this is possible in the nursing field is a matter of some contention. Carl Rogers (1967) suggested that the relationship between the one being helped and the helper *is a mutual one* in therapy and counselling. Whether or not it can be mutual between two colleagues is an interesting and debatable point.

## Commitment within defined limits

Companionship requires commitment. The companion has to be prepared to invest time and energy in the relationship. However, an important difference between the relationship between lovers and friends, and the relationship between companions and those being accompanied, is the fact that the companionship relationship has more explicit limits. In a friendship, those limits are worked out, informally and tacitly. Quite often friends do not try to define the limits of their relationship. The same can be said of the relationship between lovers.

It is interesting to reflect on the degree to which, in Campbell's terms, we really do 'care' for our colleagues: for that is the requirement of this clause of the Code of Conduct.

## Questions for reflection and discussion

1. Have you ever experienced burnout?
2. What, for you, are the most important things about caring for another person?

### References

Campbell AV (1984) *Moderated Love*. London: SPCK.

Fawcett J (1987) Diary of a disaster. *Nursing Times* **83**: 43.

Gortner SR (1977) Strategies for survival in the practical world. *American Journal of Nursing* **77**: 618–619.

Kant I (1797) *Groundwork of the Metaphysic of Morals*. Trans. Lindsay AD. New York: Library of Literal Arts.

Kingsley, CC (1885) *The Water Babies* (1976 edn). London: Garland.

Pyne R (1987) Top secret code. *Nursing Times* **83**: 42.

Rogers CR (1967) *On Becoming a Person*. London: Constable.

Shubin S (1978) Burnout: the professional hazard in nursing. *Nursing* **18**: 7.

Storlie F (1979) Burnout: the elaboration of a concept: *American Journal of Nursing* **79**: 186–193.

# CHAPTER 14

# Assisting the Development of Colleagues

*Assist professional colleagues, in the context of your own knowledge, experience and sphere of responsibility, to develop their professional competence and assist others in the care team, including informal carers, to contribute safely and to a degree appropriate to their roles.*

In considering how to assist peers and subordinates to develop professional competence it may be worth considering how we can identify or give shape to our own knowledge and experience. After all, as the statement above notes, it is from those domains (alongside our sphere of authority) that we draw the necessary skills to help others.

## Domains of knowledge

A practical method of dividing up knowledge and experience in order to understand it is to consider the following three domains: propositional knowledge, practical knowledge and experiential knowledge (Heron, 1981; Burnard, 1987). Propositional knowledge is 'textbook' knowledge – theories, facts, models and other theoretical constructions. We need such propositional knowledge in order that we may make sense of the world around us. Theories and models help us to classify things and to categorise them in such a way as to make them intelligible. They can also help us to plan for the future, for an accurate theory usually enables us to predict, with varying degrees of accuracy, what will happen next.

Practical knowledge is knowledge gained through doing. Every time we skilfully give an injection we display practical knowledge. Practical knowledge often involves psychomotor activity and manual dexterity, but it may not. An example of the demonstration of practical knowledge which does not involve psychomotor activity is the display of counselling skills. Such skills may be developed systematically through attendance on a counselling course or through the process of doing counselling. Either way, the skilled nurse-as-counsellor exhibits distinct practical knowledge every time she successfully counsels someone.

## Propositional and practical knowledge

There are important differences between propositional knowledge and practical knowledge. Propositional knowledge involves what Ryle (1949) called 'knowing that' something is the case. Thus a nurse may know that certain things are important in order to deliver a baby, without actually possessing the skills to do so! Practical knowledge, on the other hand involves what Ryle called 'knowing how'. Thus, a nurse may know how to deliver a baby and be able to carry through the process without knowing the theoretical implications of what she is doing. Clearly, it is better that we combine both propositional and practical knowledge. What we know in a theoretical sense should tie up precisely with what we do in practice

## Experiential knowledge

Experiential knowledge, on the other hand, is personal knowledge through direct encounter with a person, place or thing. Thus, before I went to America, I had a considerable amount of propositional knowledge about the place: I had pictures in my mind about how certain places looked and I knew something of the history of America. When I visited the country, however, everything I 'knew' about it previously was changed by my direct encounter with it. This, then, is experiential knowledge. Experiential knowledge is knowledge that is personal to the individual. It is gained, as is suggested by the name, through personal experience. We cannot give another person experiential knowledge, neither can we teach it to others. In recent years there has been increasing interest in the use of experiential learning methods (Kagan, 1985; Kagan et al., 1986; Burnard 1990, 1991) in nurse education. These methods are concerned precisely with the development of experiential knowledge: understanding the world through direct encounter with it. In another sense, too, much nursing skill is learned not through the school or college of nursing but by direct experience: we learn nursing by doing it.

There are, however, limits to the value of experiential knowledge just as there are limits to the value of propositional and practical knowledge. We cannot wisely rely only on our personal experience. To do this would be to limit our knowledge base in a very important sense. If we rely only on our own experience we never give attention to the thinking or practice that have been developed by countless other people in the profession. Nor do we heed the research that has been conducted in the field. What we may choose to do, however, is to test out the theories, skills and research of others for ourselves and thus combine the domains of propositional, practical and experiential knowledge.

Consideration of the above three domains of knowledge may help us to assess our own knowledge levels. When we consider our knowledge of nursing, for example, are we clear about our theoretical deficits and assets (propositional knowledge)? Can we readily identify the skills that we have and those we lack (practical knowledge)? Are we able to consider reflectively our past experience and be clear about the experience we need in the future (experiential knowledge)? If we can do all these things then we are in a stronger position to help others to develop professional competence. Without that self-assessment we are blind to our own deficiencies and competencies. That blindness may further blind us to the deficiencies and competencies of others.

Note that it is not being suggested that we have to rectify all our deficiencies before we help others. All we have to do is to identify them, to know that they are there. Armed with this knowledge we can be better equipped to notice the theoretical, practical and experiential gaps in others. Whether or not we then go on and plug our own knowledge gaps is another ethical issue! It would seem difficult to justify on any grounds that having acknowledged our ignorance or lack of expertise or experience in a particular field, we then do nothing about it. A variant of the 'golden rule' may apply here. The golden rule is that we should do unto others only that which we would have done to us. The variant, here, may be that we should only advise others about their knowledge base if we are prepared to do something about our own.

Once we are clear, then, on our own sphere of knowledge and experience we are better able to assist others. We need, also, to be clear about our 'sphere of authority' as referred to in the Code of Conduct. For most practical purposes our sphere of authority is laid out, formally, in our job description. In another sense, though, that authority is granted less formally through the process of 'custom and practice'. We gain authority to carry out certain tasks through our actually doing them. The more we continue to do them, the more they become legitimised. It would seem wise for us to take stock regularly of what it is we do in our jobs and compare what we actually do with what we are required to do. This, again, calls for the vigilant sense of awareness called for in previous chapters.

## Knowledge as power

As everyone who has ever had a secret knows, it is exciting to know something that is not common knowledge. It gives the secret-holder a sense of superiority and power. Unfortunately, some nurses feel the same about professional knowledge and may be reluctant to pass it on. They feel indispensable if they have information which other nurses do not have and this helps to increase their sense of worth. In particular, this may be linked with seniority and be used to indicate that some information is 'special' to senior staff despite the fact that it could be understood by anyone and may be vital to the intelligent care of patients in a specific setting. The Code does not recognise the need for this type of retention of knowledge.

In helping others to develop, it is essential, first, that we listen to them and try to enter their 'frame of reference' – their view of the world. The great temptation is to imagine that everyone views the world as we do. The truth is, of course, that we all view the same or similar situations quite differently. Such perceptual differences may be accounted for by the fact of our differences of physiology, background, upbringing, culture, education and personality. We have also lived unique lives and experienced the world as no other person. Given these individual differences, it is vital that we learn to listen to the other person carefully, for it is only through such intense listening that we can hope to enter into the frame of reference of the other person.

## Counselling skills training

Many courses are now available in colleges and extra-mural departments that offer basic counselling skills. Almost all such courses emphasise the need for accurate listening and offer exercises for the development of the art and skill of listening. Basic listening and attending skills are also being introduced into nurse training programmes. In psychiatric nursing, such skills are seen as essential and prescribed by the 1982 syllabus of training (ENB, 1982). Whether through basic nurse training or through attendance at a course of training, it is recommended that all nurses undergo some sort of listening skills training.

If such formal training is not available, individuals can do much to sharpen up their skills on their own. One very simple exercise is merely to sit with a friend or colleague and pay full attention to what he is saying. This involves temporarily 'suspending judgment' or being critical of what he is saying: the aim is purely to hear what is said. Such an exercise constitutes part of what Heron (1973) calls 'conscious use of self'. By this is meant the constant choosing of a particular type of behaviour (in this case, listening) rather than merely letting our behaviour 'happen'. We can train ourselves to be more effective listeners and the conscious effort involved can mean that we understand others more clearly.

Once we have heard the other person, we can help him to assess his own needs in terms of professional competence. It is worth noting the emphasis made by the Code of Conduct: we are requested to assist peers '. . . in accordance with their needs'. Note that it is not our perception of their needs – the needs are to be defined by the person concerned. Thus we need to develop skills in helping others to identify their own needs. This can be done through the process of listening, described above, and through the use of questions that encourage the other person to problem solve. Such questions can be aimed at encouraging the other person to identify gaps in their knowledge or skill. Examples of such questions may be:

1. What do you need to learn next?
2. What sort of information may help you now?
3. Can you identify the nursing procedures that you carry out effectively and those that you are not so sure about?
4. Or, simply, 'what do you need to do next?'

In each of the above cases, it is the individual, herself, who is responsible for identifying areas for further development, whether in the domain of professional, practical or experiential knowledge. Such an approach is quite in keeping with progressive approaches to education and training which stress a student-centred approach (Rogers, 1983; Knowles, 1978, 1981). If we are to encourage our patients to develop autonomy and to take part in planning part of their care, it is reasonable that nurses develop their own skill and knowledge levels through this student-centred approach.

F

## Post-Registration Education and Practice Project

Following on from the recommendations of Project 2000, the UKCC has turned its attention to the nurse's need for continuing education and issued their proposals in 1991. The recommendations are concerned with the needs of nurses in clinical practice (a separate document *Report on Proposals for the Future of Community Education and Practice* deals with nurses working outside institutional settings). Full details can be found by reading the reports. However, one of the important proposals is that newly qualified nurses should have guidance from a more senior nurse or mentor. This fits in well with the requirement that nurses should be prepared to help colleagues develop their professional role and skills. The knowledge gained by practical experience is also recognised and is accorded credit when more formal qualification is sought.

## Questions for reflection and discussion

1. In what ways do you use your own 'practical and experiential knowledge'?
2. Are you aware of the *limits* of your knowledge?

### References

Burnard P (1987) Towards an epistemological basis for experiential learning in nurse education. *Journal of Advanced Nursing* **12**: 189–193.

Burnard P (1990) *Learning Human Skills: an Experiential Guide for Nurses.* Oxford: Butterworth-Heinemann.

Burnard P (1991) *Experiential Learning in Action.* Aldershot: Avebury.

ENB (1982) *Syllabus of Training: Professional Register. Part 3: (Registered Mental Nurse).* London and Cardiff: English and Welsh National Boards for Nursing, Midwifery and Health Visiting.

Heron J (1973) *Experiential Training Techniques*: Human Potential Research Project. Guildford: University of Surrey.

Heron J (1981) Philosophical basis for a new paradigm. In: Reason P and Rowan J (eds) *Human Inquiry: a Sourcebook of New Paradigm Research.* Chichester: Wiley.

Kagan C (ed) (1985) *Interpersonal Skills in Nursing: Research and Applications.* London: Croom Helm.

Kagan C, Evans J and Kay B (1986) *A Manual of Interpersonal Skills for Nurses: an Experiential Approach.* London: Harper and Row.

Knowles M (1978) *The Adult Learner: a neglected species.* 2nd edn. Texas: Gulf.

Knowles M (1981) *The Modern Practice of Adult Education.* 2nd edn. Chicago: Follett.

Rogers CR (1983) *Freedom to Learn for the Eighties*. Columbus, Ohio: Merrill.
Ryle G (1949) *The Concept of Mind*. Harmondsworth: Peregrine.

# CHAPTER 15

# Rewards

*Refuse any gift, favour or hospitality from patients or clients currently in your care which might be interpreted as seeking to exert influence to obtain preferential consideration.*

A great deal of energy is exerted in trying to find out why nurses leave the profession often very soon after qualifying. While the answer to this question is obviously important perhaps it is surprising that any stay. Not only does the nurse work unsocial hours and undertake hard physical work but she spends the day with people who are at their least attractive due to illness, pain and distress. Nevertheless many nurses spend all their working lives in the profession and would not consider doing anything else. Even though rates of pay have improved in recent years they are not sufficiently attractive to be the main reason why these nurses are happy in their work.

All people seek satisfaction in their daily life and this can be provided in a number of ways. It is quite common to talk about 'meeting the patient's needs' but nurses also have needs and it is the way in which these are or are not met that decides whether or not they remain in the profession.

## Social exchange

This meeting of needs is of course not restricted to nurses, and social anthropologists have described it as a form of 'social exchange'. Cynics argue that little is done in the world from purely altruistic motives but that in every activity there is a reward of some sort. While some aspects of social exchange have a complex economic connotation, other aspects appear to be important for their symbolic value and the social ties that they create. For example, Malinowski (1922), states that there is a:

> Fundamental human impulse to display, to share, to bestow; the deep tendency to create social ties through the exchange of gifts . . . giving for the sake of giving is one of the most important features of Trobriand society and, from its very general and fundamental nature, I submit it is a universal feature of all primitive societies.

A more recent writer, Levi-Strauss (1969), points out that even in Western society there is a strong feeling towards reciprocity which extends to invitations, Christmas cards and birthday presents; all of which by their exchange indicate social ties between giver and recipient. Gouldner (1969) also develops this idea and states that 'it would seem that there can be stable patterns of reciprocity "qua" exchange only in so far as each party has both rights and duties'.

Homans (1961) considers that the process of exchange will only continue if the participants derive some benefit from it.

> The open secret of human exchange is to give to the other man behaviour that is more valuable to him than it is costly to you and to get from him behaviour that is more valuable to you than it is costly to him.

The position of health care within the UK is such that it is frequently considered 'free' because payment is not made at the point of delivery. So with nursing care, many patients feel that they get more care than that which is paid for by either their insurance contributions or by the salary that the nurse receives. Thus there is an interesting relationship where the nurse may be seen as a giver of a gift, her care, and the patient as the receiver of the gift without the normal provision for the return of gifts.

Indeed there is no equality in the relationship of nurse and patient at the time that care is being given. Although the patient may only be in a state of temporary dependence, in the case of the chronic sick, handicapped or dying the dependence may be permanent. Therefore it may be considered that repayment for nursing care is impossible. It is this inequality of relationship that places nursing in the category of occupations which are considered vocational by the general public and which gives nurses much of their esteem. An effort to restore this balance is frequently made by the patient by the gift of gratitude.

However, in view of the reasons why individuals take up nursing it may be that they are repaid in that the dependence of the patient satisfies the nurse's psychological needs. Nurses themselves tend to indicate that this is the case and if not prevented may prolong the patient's dependency.

## Creative altruism

Titmuss (1970) calls this activity 'creative altruism', creative in the sense that the self is realised with the help of others. In discussing blood donors, he says that giving blood 'allows the biological need to help to express itself'. Tonnies (1887) (in Loomis, 1955) sees such activity more cynically saying '*Do,utdes*', 'What I do for you, I do only as a means to effect your simultaneous, previous or later service for me. . . . To get something from you is my end, my service is thereto which I contribute unwillingly'.

Maybe this sort of statement throws light on the fact that care of some classes of patients is seen as less prestigious in the eyes of society, which tends to classify the worth of individuals in relation to the contribution that they are able to make to society. It is not difficult to see that the stigma of dependency rests most heavily on the old, the chronically sick, the mentally handicapped and those who are unlikely to be able to recover and make a contribution to society. This stigmatisation may also rest on those who care for these people and may account for the fact that those who consider nursing a vocation may choose to work with these groups. Pinker (1971) has described this situation, where the individual is unlikely to be able to repay, as one where the person is subject to a 'comparison gap'. Furthermore, he points out that the relationship between the giver and the receiver is always inherently an instable and unequal one and that although gratitude may be used to help to restore the balance, because the gift was given first the gratitude may be given with a sense of coercion. Money is the commodity which produces instant equivalence.

Social exchange in this context may be most easily depicted as a balance: on one side are the nurse's needs and on the other side the satisfactions provided by caring for clients, see Table 15.1.

Obviously different nurses have different emphases relating to these needs. Some have a great need to provide physical care, others have a great thirst for knowledge and so on. Most meet their needs by working in the area that provides the greatest opportunity to match their needs with those of the patient. A nurse getting most satisfaction from physical care will be likely to work with long-stay, continuing care patients. Those with a desire

| Nurse's needs | Patient's needs |
|---|---|
| Knowledge | Information |
| To give physical care | Physical care |
| To develop skills | Psychological and spiritual care |
| Have contented patients | |

**Table 15.1** Meeting the nurse's needs

to increase their knowledge of medical science will seek work in acute units, possible intensive care.

Patients rarely appreciate this situation and frequently say 'how can I repay you nurse?' little realising that the very fact that they are in the role of patient makes it possible for the role of nurse to exist. All this would indicate that the interaction between nurse and patient must inevitably produce feelings of stigma on behalf of the patient and it is to overcome this discomfort that some patients may offer the nurse a gift, either in kind or money.

While verbal gratitude is greatly welcomed by nurses and indeed Stockwell (1976) found that nurses felt that it was their right, the giving of gifts to express gratitude is more contentious. Many health authorities have a policy stating that individuals must not receive gifts from patients and if a patient wishes to express gratitude in this way, then the gift must be given either to the unit or the authority via the administration. The reason for such a policy is easy to appreciate as it would be very easy for such a gift to be given as a bribe to ensure preferential treatment and the Code is very clear in its statement that the nurse must 'refuse to accept any gift, favour or hospitality which might be interpreted as seeking to exert undue influence to obtain preferential consideration'.

While most nurses are well aware of the dangers of accepting a gift which might be interpreted as a bribe from a patient, they are perhaps less sensitive to the gifts offered by pharmaceutical or other firms. In this they are not alone, the medical profession frequently accepts hospitality from such sources. The question has to be asked, does the acceptance of a diary or the sponsorship of a conference from a commercial firm put me or my organisation under any sort of pressure to buy from that firm in preference to any other? If the answer is 'yes' then the offer of help, in whatever form, must be refused. If there is no pressure, not even a moral one, then it may be permissible to accept the offer. However, the relationship is always a potentially dangerous one.

In the present social setting when there is great competition for

Health Service contracts the nurse has to be extremely careful not to get involved, even if unwittingly in an activity which may constitute bribery or unfair practice.

## Questions for reflection and discussion

1. In what circumstances do you feel you might be tempted to accept a 'reward'?
2. Are you rewarded for what you do as a nurse?

## References

Chapman CM (1984) *Theory of Nursing: Practical Application*. London: Harper and Row.
Gouldner AW (1969) The norm of reciprocity, a preliminary statement. *American Sociological Review* **28**: 169.
Henderson V (1962) *Basic Principles of Nursing Care*. Switzerland: ICN.
Homans GC (1961) *Social Behaviour in its Elementary Forms*. New York: Harcourt, Brace and World.
Levi-Strauss C (1969) *The Elementary Structures of Kinship*. Boston: Beacon Press.
Loomis P (1955 translation) *Community and Associations*. London: Routledge and Kegan Paul.
Malinowski B (1922) *Argonauts of the Western Pacific*. New York: Routledge and Kegan Paul.
Pinker R (1971) *Social Theory and Social Policy*. London: Heinemann.
Stockwell F (1976) *The Unpopular Patient*. London: Royal College of Nursing.
Titmus R (1970) *The Gift Relationship*. London: Allen and Unwin.

# CHAPTER 16

# Advertising

*Ensure that your registration status is not used in the promotion of commercial products or services, declare any financial and other interests in relevant organisations providing such goods and services and ensure that your professional judgment is not influenced by any commercial considerations.*

Professional nurses are constantly asked by members of the general public, neighbours and friends for advice on health matters. This is inevitable and can be seen as part of the nurse's responsibility to society. Part of this advice may involve the nurse in offering her opinion on what medicine to take for a cough or how to feed a baby. In offering this advice it is likely that the nurse will mention a trade name. It is doubtful whether such advice could be considered as advertising. However manufacturing firms may wish to have a professional nurse endorse their products either overtly by appearing in an advertisement or covertly by accepting free or cheap samples of products which may then be passed on to patients or clients. It is this type of activity that is referred to in the final phrase of the Code of Conduct.

## Advertising

Advertising is an activity in which the person who is the object of the advertisement is persuaded to act in a particular way. It may in fact be considered as a specific form of propaganda. There have been many studies to ascertain how propaganda works. A study by Katz and Lazarsfeld (1955) identified people who acted as 'opinion leaders'. These were those whose opinions were sort by friends, neighbours and acquaintances. In the area of public affairs these people tended to be of a higher social class than those seeking advice.

The medium used is also important, Lazarsfeld et al. (1944) showed that personal influence was much more effective than any other form of communication in producing change. Influence therefore is likely to flow down from opinion leaders, by word of mouth, to the recipients.

Peake (1955) found that the effectiveness of information on attitude change was related to the importance of the outcome of the information on the individual. There are few areas of life that are more important to an individual than those which affect the health of them or their family. Therefore these studies are important when considering the role that may be played by professional health carers in formulating public opinion.

Nurses, midwives and health visitors are held in very great respect by the public who credit them with a high degree of knowledge and also accord to them a high level of trust. In addition they are people who normally have personal contact with the patients. Because of this any product recommended by a nurse is likely to be purchased. This places a great responsibility on the shoulders of the nurse and it is vital that any recommendation is based on the best possible knowledge, and is unbiased.

Obviously if a nurse has received payment in order to sponsor a specific product then he or she may well feel that product is the one that should be used and/or recommended even though in some cases another product would be more suitable. It is because of the danger of bias affecting professional judgment that the final phrase states that a registered nurse, midwife and health visitor shall 'avoid the use of professional qualifications in the promotion of commercial products in order not to compromise the independent professional judgment on which patients/clients rely'.

## Code of Conduct

Following the publication of the Code of Professional Conduct there were many questions received at the UKCC by nurses who wished to become or remain involved in advertising. In an attempt to explain and elaborate the intention of the Code, the UKCC issued a separate publication covering advertising (UKCC, 1985). In this document there is explanation of when and how the nurse, midwife and health visitor may be involved in using a professional qualification and not be guilty of professional misconduct, and which situations are to be avoided. It describes the following situations:

1. Advertising for professional work is allowed providing that such an advertisement is not ostentatious and does not imply that the practitioner is to be preferred over others. This advertisement may be for general work or be for work in some speciality, in which case it is permissible to state the fact that the practitioner has completed a specialist course and has a recorded qualification.
2. A nurse, midwife or health visitor who owns or manages a business associated with professional practice (for example a nursing home) may use the appropriate qualifications in advertisements for that business or on letter headings, etc.
3. A nurse, midwife or health visitor employed by another person or business which requires her to call on other health care professionals or institutions to promote products may use the appropriate qualifications on visiting cards or other stationery.
4. Nurses, midwives and health visitors may be involved in providing advice for writing or featuring in promotional literature or films associated with commercial products. In this case the appearance of the professional's name in the credits should not be accompanied by the qualification status. However if the production is for educational or documentary purposes and could not be considered in any way as advertising then the registration status may be stated. In addition the practitioner may use registration qualifications in association with participation in conferences and in radio or television programmes providing that such participation cannot be seen to be a way of advertising the practitioner.
5. Advertising for professional work outside nursing, midwifery or health visiting, i.e. within the province of another profession, should not be undertaken if that other profession does not allow its practitioners to advertise. If the other profession does allow advertising and the registered nurse, midwife or health visitor wishes to use their registered qualification, advice and permission should first be obtained from the UKCC.

This guidance document, which is not quoted in full in this chapter, should be consulted by any registered nurse, midwife or health visitor who is in any doubt regarding her proposed action.

To summarise, attitude change is most likely to occur when the person presenting the information is of a higher social class than those receiving the message, is in a position of trust, and is able to give the information verbally.

As stated elsewhere the registered nurse practitioner has a special place in society. The possession of a registered qualification implies not only the achievement of specific skills and knowledge but also the holding of specific values and attitudes. This privileged status offered to members of the caring professions must not be abused and this may require a high standard of behaviour in all areas of life. Most professionals accept this and act accordingly, however not all are sufficiently aware of the effect that the use of their qualifications may have when linked with commercial products. In a similar way not all are sensitive to the restraint that may be placed upon them by the acceptance of gifts or hospitality from commercial firms.

## Questions for reflection and discussion

1. Do you feel in any way limited by this element of the Code?
2. Should nurses be free to advertise their professional expertise?

## References

Katz D and Lazarsfeld PF (1955) *Personal Influence: the Part Played by People in the Flow of Mass Communication*. Glencoe, Ill: Free Press.
Lazarsfeld PF, Berelson B and Gaudet H (1944) *The People's Choice*. New York: Duell, Sloan & Pearce.
Peake H (1955) Attitude and motivation. In: Jones MR (ed) *Nebraska Symposium on Motivation*. Lincoln: University Nebraska Press.
UKCC (1985) *Advertising by Registered Nurses, Midwives and Health Visitors*. London: UKCC.

# CHAPTER 17

# Conclusion

In the preceding chapters we have explored a variety of theories and practical approaches to ethical and professional issues in nursing. In one sense, how we decide to act in a nursing situation is determined for us by the Code of Conduct. The Code lays down broad principles and offers a framework to guide professional action. What we as individuals have to do, however, is to interpret those principles and very often we have to decide for ourselves what to do. Again, this book has offered some pointers to how such decisions may be made. The book cannot make those decisions. Nor can it account for the many and varied situations that arise in everyday nursing practice that are 'exceptions to the rule'. After all, in real life, situations are rarely experienced as they are printed in books!

In closing, it may be worth reconsidering some of the ways of making ethical and professional decisions that have been alluded to in this book. First, we may appeal to a code of conduct as a means of decision-making. Clearly, as this book is about such a code, it is felt that codes can be useful means of helping and guiding in the decision-making process. There are, of course, other codes that can be referred to, the most notable being particular ethical codes as outlined within specific religious sects. We have noted, too, that atheists and agnostics may also have codes to which they refer.

## Conscience

Another means of making ethical and professional decisions is through considerations of conscience. Freud called the person's conscience their 'superego' and argued that the development of such a conscience or superego evolved out of the internalisation of parental values, beliefs and attitudes at an early age (Hall, 1954). Thus, when we appeal to our conscience it is as though we were experiencing one or both of our parents 'looking over our shoulder' as we make a particular decision. Another way of viewing the development of conscience is to see it in terms of socialisation. As a person grows and develops through life he absorbs and learns the particular set of beliefs and values of his parents and also takes account of the broader set of beliefs and values of the particular culture in which he grows up. This process of socialisation must clearly affect decision-making. Decisions are not made in isolation nor are they made outside the particular culture in which the decision-maker lives.

This notion of culture-bound ethical and professional decisions is an important one. It is tempting to believe that the beliefs and values of 'our' culture are the 'right' ones. Clearly, different cultures produce different values and different values will be reflected in different sorts of ethical and professional decisions, made in different countries and societies.

## Utilitarianism

Another approach to ethical and professional decision-making is via the notion of utilitarianism – arguing that what is good and right is that which creates the greatest happiness for the greatest number. Indeed, many decisions are made on this basis but we may want to ponder on (a) who decides what is likely to create the greatest good? and (b) what happens to those that are not contained within the 'greatest number'?

It may be worth considering, too, Sartre's (1956, 1973) notion of 'situational ethics'. In order to understand this notion, it is important to consider, also, the theory of existentialism, for which Sartre was famous.

## Existentialism

Existentialism, as an approach to philosophy, may be encapsulated by Sartre's famous epigram that 'existence comes prior to essence' (Sartre, 1973, p. 26). In order to understand this, it may be useful to look at an example that Sartre, himself, uses. If we consider a man-made object such as a paperknife, we can realise that before it came into existence, someone sat down and designed it. For the paperknife, then, its 'essence' came prior to its 'existence': before it was made, someone had a fair idea of what it was going to be for. Sartre argues that, for people, exactly the opposite is true. First of all we exist, then we create our essence. Thus there is no one 'designing' us before we exist: we start from nothing and then we are responsible for what we become.

Contained in Sartre's argument is the notion that people are (psychologically, at least) free to choose how they view themselves and the world. The temptation, very often, is for people to blame the past, other people or circumstances for how they are today. While these factors clearly have an influence, Sartre is saying that today the individual decides for himself: he can choose to blame the past or circumstances, but that does not change his personal responsibility for decision-making. A person is what he makes himself. Clearly, as we have noted, this is a psychological freedom – a freedom of thought. We cannot exercise a similar physical or social freedom. It would be ludicrous, for instance, to argue that a person could choose to be seven foot tall or that he could choose the social circumstances into which he was born! The point Sartre is making is that, given those physical and social limitations, people are makers of their own destiny.

It may be noted at this point, that while Sartre's view of existentialism is atheistic this need not necessarily be the case. Other commentators have argued for a Christian existentialism (Macquarrie, 1966). This version argues that while God was the prime mover, it is man who still has to decide on his own future and make his own decisions. In this version, man has been given 'free will' by God. In Sartre's version, God does not exist in the first place: man has free will anyway.

The second issue is the individual's responsibility for his life and his decision-making. A person cannot be free and yet not responsible. Imagine, for instance, that I say 'I am free to get married and I have chosen to do so, but the decision is really my parents'.' Such a statement is plainly illogical. Clearly, if I am free to choose, I cannot make another person responsible for my choice otherwise no such 'choice' exists.

These factors have important repercussions for ethical and professional decision-making. If Sartre's position is accepted (and it may not be), then the responsibility for all decisions rests squarely with the individual.

It may be worth considering to what degree nursing situations can be clarified through an appeal to situational ethics. Clearly in many situations the nurse is dependent upon others to share in making decisions. Nor may we be keen to take on board Sartre's notion of total responsibility.

Such argument can, however, make the nurse aware of how important ethical and behavioural decisions are and how important it is for her to shoulder responsibility. Such argument can also awaken nurses to the importance of considering the context of ethical decision-making. While the Code of Conduct can be used as a guide to such decisions, it must also be borne in mind that this situation, for this person, is unique. It is necessary to remain flexible and open-minded and, where possible, come to each situation afresh. In weighing up the pros and cons of any situation and relating them to prior experience and knowledge, it must also be acknowledged how different this new situation is.

Perhaps, however, Sartre's position is a little black and white. It may be argued that many ethical and professional decisions are made by considering the evidence and comparing that evidence with previous situations that have occurred and with which this situation may be compared. Out of this consideration and reflection on past experience arises the 'new' decision. An example may be useful here. If a nurse manager is attempting to make an important decision about how best to advise a member of staff she may well reflect back on previous situations which mirror this one, consider the 'unique' features of the present situation and look for some sort of 'fit' between past and present experience. Out of this balanced view, the manager makes her decision. In one sense, she is of course alone in making that decision. In another sense, however, she has considerable precedent, in terms of her own and other people's past experience, on which to draw. Decisions are never made in isolation. As has been discussed throughout this book, they arise out of a wide range of cultural, social, psychological and personal contexts. Perhaps, then, 'unique' situations are not as unique as they first appear!

One particular theme has recurred frequently throughout this book: the notion of the 'golden rule'. This is usually expressed as the idea that we should treat others as we ourselves would wish to be treated. This would seem to be a necessary requirement of anyone who makes ethical and professional decisions. The notion marks out the importance of fundamental human considerations: respect for others, consideration of the possible consequences of action, and the need always to treat people as subjects and never as objects. Without such fundamental considerations, it seems difficult to see how any notion of ethical or professional decisions can begin to be made. It is notable, however, that even the 'golden rule' has its limitations. It may work well enough all the time that the individual is a thoughtful, caring person who wishes, themselves, to be treated that way. It does not account for the person who does not care how they are treated! In this case, clearly, the notion of treating others as you would wish to be treated, does not apply! Christians would, of course, quote a higher authority for this type of action, the words of Jesus, 'This is my commandment, that ye love one another. . .' (John 15, 12).

This book offers a variety of ways of addressing ethical and professional issues. The subject is a complex one and we hope that the book has raised more questions than it has answered. There cannot be a ready guide to the sorts of issues discussed in this book nor can there be a consensus on how to make decisions. What all ethical and professional decisions require is a firm grasp of as many of the facts as possible, an understanding of the various philosophical and theoretical ways of addressing problems of this nature plus a certain courage and determination to make decisions. This is true throughout the field of nursing, from nurse learner to the most senior administrator or educator. Nursing is necessarily about decision-making.

Ethics and professional practice are constantly changing. Just as Project 2000 and the changes in nursing practice have changed the way that nursing is taught and organised, so those changes will bring about the need to view new situations in different ways. The important thing about the ideas in this book is that they offer *ways of thinking* about situations, contexts and people. What can never be offered is a final, authoritative book which tells you 'how to do it'. The important thing, as a nurse, is to develop as and remain a *reflective practitioner*: a person who thinks and reflects about what he or she does and then acts *knowingly*.

### References

Hall C (1954) *A Primer of Freudian Psychology*. New York: Basic Books.
Macquarrie J (1966) *Studies in Christian Existentialism*. London: SCM.
Sartre J-P (1956) *Being and Nothingness: an Essay on Phenomenological Ontology*. Translated by H Barnes. New York: Philosophical Library.
Sartre J-P (1973) *Existentialism and Humanism*. Translated by P Mairet. London: Methuen.

# Recommended Further Reading

Aroskar MA (1980a) Anatomy of an ethical dilemma: the theory, the practice. *American Journal of Nursing* **80**(4) 658–663.

Aroskar MA (1980b) Ethics of nurse–patient relationships. *Nurse Educator* **5**(2) 18–20.

Atwood AH (1979) The mentor in clinical practice. *Nursing Outlook* **27**: 714–717.

Austin R (1978) Professionalism and the nature of nursing reward. *Journal of Advanced Nursing* **3**: 19–23.

Baly M (1984) *Professional Responsibility*. 2nd edn. Chichester: Wiley.

Barker P (1989) Reflections on the philosophy of caring in mental health. *International Journal of Nursing Studies* **26**(2) 131–141.

Barnes HE (1967) *An Existential Ethics*. New York: Knopf.

Bartley WW (1971) *Morality and Religion*. London: Macmillan.

Baruth LG (1987) *An Introduction to the Counselling Profession*. Englewood Cliffs, New Jersey: Prentice Hall.

Beardshaw V (1981) *Conscientious Objectors at Work*. London: Social Audit Ltd.

Beauchamp TL and Walter L (1978) *Contemporary Issues in Bioethics*. Encino, California: Dickenson.

Beck CM, Crittenden BS and Sullivan EV (eds) (1971) *Moral Education*. Toronto: Toronto University Press.

Benjamin M and Curtis J (1981) *Ethics in Nursing*. New York: OUP.

Benner P and Wrubel J (1989) *The Primacy of Caring: Stress and Coping in Health and Illness*. Menlo Park, California: Addison-Wesley.

Benner P (1984) *From Novice to Expert: Excellence and Power in Clinicial Nursing Practice*. Menlo Park, California: Addison-Wesley.

Bergman R (1976) Evolving ethical concepts for nursing. *International Nursing Review* **23**(4) 116–117.

Berry C (1987) *The Rites of Life: Christians and Bio-Medical Decision Making*. London: Hodder and Stoughton.

Blackham HJ (1968) *Humanism*. Harmondsworth: Pelican.

Blomquist C, Veatch RM and Fenner D (1975) The teaching of medical ethics. *Journal of Medical Ethics* **1**(2) 96–103.

Bluglass R (1983) *A Guide to the Mental Health Act 1983*. Edinburgh: Churchill Livingstone.

Bok S (1980) *Lying: Moral Choice in Public and Private Life*. London: Quartet.

Brazier M (1987) *Medicine, Patients and the Law*. Harmondsworth: Pelican.

Bridges W (1973) The three faces of humanistic education. In: Orlosky DE and Smith, BO (eds) *Curriculum Development: Issues and Insights*. Chicago: Rand McNally.

British Medical Association (1980) *Handbook of Medical Ethics*. London: BMA.

Broad CD (1930) *Five Types of Ethical Theory*. London: Routledge and Kegan Paul.

Brody JK (1988) Virtue ethics, caring and nursing. *Scholarly Inquiry for Nursing Practice: An International Journal* 2(2) 87–96.

Campbell AV (1984a) *Moral Dilemmas in Medicine*. 3rd edn. Edinburgh: Churchill Livingstone.

Carper BA (1979) The ethics of caring. *Advances in Nursing Science* 1(3) 11–19.

Cash K (1990) Nursing models and the idea of nursing. *International Journal of Nursing Studies* 27(3) 249–256.

Chapman CM (1977) Concepts of professionalism. *Journal of Advanced Nursing* 2: 51–55.

Chene A (1983) The concept of autonomy in adult education: a philosophical discussion. *Adult Education Quarterly* 32(1) 38–47.

Christie RJ and Hoffmaster CB (1986) *Ethical Issues in Family Medicine*. New York: Oxford University Press.

Churchill L (1977) Ethical issues of a profession in transition. *American Journal of Nursing* 77(5) 873–875.

Clay T (1987) *Nurses: Power and Politics*. London: Heinemann.

Davis CM (1981) Affective education for the health profession. *Physical Therapy* 61(11): 1587–1593.

Davis BD (ed) (1983) *Research into Nurse Education*. London: Croom Helm.

Davis AJ and Aroskar MA (1983) *Ethical Dilemmas and Nursing Practice*. Norwalk, Connecticut: Appleton-Century-Crofts.

Davis B (ed) (1987) *Nursing Education: Research and Developments*. London: Croom Helm.

Downie RS and Calman KC (1987) *Healthy Respect: Ethics in Health Care*. London: Faber and Faber.

Doxiadis S (ed) (1987) *Ethical Dilemmas in Health Promotion*. Chichester: Wiley.

Dryden W, Charles-Edwards and Woolfe R (1989) *Handbook of Counselling in Britain*. London: Routledge and Kegan Paul.

Ededel A (1955) *Ethical Judgement*. New York: Free Press.

Etzioni A (1969) *The Semi-Professions and Their Organisation*. New York: Free Press.

Evans B (1984) *Freedom to Choose*. London: The Bodley Head.

Famighetti RA (1981) Experiential learning: the close encounters of the institutional kind. *Gerontology and Geriatric Education* 2(2) 129–132.

Faulder C (1985) *Whose Body is It? The Troubling Issue of Informed Consent*. London: Virago.

Field D (1984) 'We didn't want him to die on his own'. Nurses' accounts of nursing dying patients. *Journal of Advanced Nursing* 9: 59–70.

General Medical Council (1983) *Professional Conduct and Discipline; Fitness to Practice*. London: GMC.

Gibson RL and Mitchell MH (1986) *Introduction to Counselling and Guidance*. London: Collier Macmillan.

Gillon R (1986) *Philosophical Medical Ethics*. Chichester: Wiley.

Hall J (1990) Towards a psychology of caring. *British Journal of Clinical Psychology* **29**: 129–144.

Hamrick M and Stone C (1979) Promoting experiential learning. *Health Education* **10**(4) 38–41.

Haring B (1974) *Medical Ethics*. Slough: St Paul Publications.

Harris J (1986) *The Value of Life: An Introduction to Medical Ethics*. London: Routledge and Kegan Paul.

Harrison LL (1990) Maintaining the ethic of caring in nursing. *Journal of Advanced Nursing* **15**: 125–127.

Hirst PH (1974) *Moral Education in a Secular Society*. London: University of London Press.

Horan F and Jackson V (1984) Abortion: who decides? *Nursing Times* **80**(10) 16–18.

Jarvis P (1983) *The Theory and Practice of Adult and Continuing Education*. London: Croom Helm.

Jarvis P (1977) Some comments on the RCN Code of Professional Conduct. *Nursing Mirror* **145**(47) 27–28.

Jarvis P (1983) Religiosity: a theoretical analysis of the human response to the problem of meaning. Institute for the Study of Worship and Religious Architecture, *Research Bulletin*: 51–66.

Jarvis P (1985) *The Sociology of Adult and Continuing Education*. London: Croom Helm.

Jarvis P (1987) Meaningful and meaningless experience: towards an understanding of learning from life. *Adult Education Quarterly* **37**: 3.

Jeffrey R (1979) Normal rubbish: deviant patients in casualty departments. *Sociology of Health and Illness* **1**(1) 90–107.

Johnson M (1983) Ethics in nurse education: a comment. *Nurse Education Today* **3**: 58–59.

Jupe M (1987) Ethics and nursing practice. *Senior Nurse* **7**(3) 49–51.

Kemp J (1970) *Ethical Naturalism*. London: Macmillan.

Kennedy I (1981) *Unmasking Medicine*. London: Allen and Unwin.

Kilty J (1987) Staff Development for Nurse Education: Practitioners Supporting Students: A Report of a 5-Day Development Workshop. *Human Potential Research Project*. Guildford: University of Surrey.

King EC (1984) *Affective Education in Nursing: A Guide to Teaching and Assessment*. Maryland: Aspen.

Kirschenbaum H (1977) *Advanced Values Clarification*. La Jolla, California: University Associates.

Kitson AL (1987) A comparative analysis of lay caring and professional caring relationships. *International Journal of Nursing Studies* **24**(2) 155–165.

Kleinig J (1985) *Ethical Issues in Psychosurgery*. London: Allen and Unwin.

Kleinman A (1988) *The Illness Narratives: Suffering, Healing and the Human Condition*. New York: Basic Books.

Knight M and Field D (1981) Silent conspiracy: coping with dying cancer patients on acute surgical wards. *Journal of Advanced Nursing* **6**: 221–229.

Kottler JA and Brown RW (1985) *Introduction to Therapeutic Counselling.* Monterey, California: Brooks-Cole.

Larson PJ (1984) Important nurse caring behaviours perceived by patients with cancer. *Oncology Nursing Forum* **11**(6) 46–50.

Lazarus RS and Folkman S (1984) *Stress, Appraising and Coping.* New York: Springer.

Legge D (1982) *The Education of Adults in Britain.* Milton Keynes: Open University Press.

Leininger MM (ed) (1981) *Caring: An Essential Human Need.* New Jersey: Charles B. Slack.

Leininger MM (1988) History, issues, and trends in the discovery and uses of care in nursing. In: Leininger MM (ed) *Care: Discovery and Uses in Clinical and Community Nursing.* Detroit: Wayne State University Press, 11–28.

Levine M (1977) Ethics: nursing ethics and the ethical nurse. *American Journal of Nursing* **77**(5) 845–849.

Lewin K (1952) *Field Theory and Social Change.* London: Tavistock.

Llewelyn S (1984) The cost of giving: emotional growth and emotional stress. In: Skevington S (ed) *Understanding Nurses: the Social Psychology of Nursing.* Chichester: Wiley, 49–645.

Llewelyn SP (1989) Caring: the cost to nurses and relatives. In: Broome AK (ed) *Health Psychology: Processes and Applications.* London: Chapman and Hall, 114–129.

Lorber J (1975) Good patients and problem patients: conformity and deviance in a general hospital. *Journal of Health and Social Behaviour* **16**(2) 213–225.

Magee B (1978) *Men of Ideas: Some Creators of Contemporary Philosophy.* London: BBC.

McGilloway O and Myco F (eds) (1985) *Nursing and Spiritual Care.* London: Harper and Row.

Melia K (1984) Cracking the new code. *Nursing Times* **80**(43) 20.

Meyers DW (1970) *The Human Body and the Law.* Edinburgh: Edinburgh University Press.

Mezeiro J (1981) A critical theory of adult learning and education. *Adult Education* **32**(1) 3–24.

Mill JS (1910) *Utilitarianism, Liberty and Representative Government.* London: Dent.

Moore D (1987) The buck stops with you. *Nursing Times* **83**(39) 54–56.

Moore GE (1903) *Principia Ethica.* London: Cambridge University Press.

Morris C (1956) *Varieties of Human Value.* Chicago: University of Chicago Press.

Neuberger J (1987) *Caring for People of Different Faiths.* London: Austin Cornish.

Niblett WR (1963) *Moral Education in a Changing Society.* London: Faber and Faber.

Niebuhr H (1977) *Revitalizing American Education: a New Approach that Might Just Work.* Belmont, California: Wadsworth.

Nightingale F (1974) *Notes on Nursing: what it is and what it is not* (new edn). London: Blackie.

Nutall P (1982) Take me to your mentor. *Nursing Times* **78**(20) 826.

Nyberg D (ed) (1975) *The Philosophy of Open Education*. London: Routledge and Kegan Paul.

Papper S (1983) *Doing Right: Everyday Medical Ethics*. Boston: Little, Brown.

Partridge KB (1978) Nursing values in a changing society. *Nursing Outlook* **26**(6) 356–360.

Paterson JB and Zderad LT (1988) *Humanistic Nursing*. New York: National League for Nursing. (Originally published in 1976).

Patka F (ed) (1972) *Existential Thinkers and Thought*. Secaucus, New Jersey: Citadel Press.

Paton HJ (1969) *The Moral Law: Kant's Groundwork of the Metaphysics of Morals*. London: Hutchinson.

Phillips M and Dawson J (1985) *Doctors' Dilemmas: Medical Ethics and Contemporary Science*. Brighton, Sussex: Harvester Press.

Pyne R (1980) *Professional Discipline in Nursing*. London: Blackwell.

Pyne R (1987) A professional duty to shout. *Nursing Times* **83**(42) 30–31.

RCN (1977) *Ethics Related to Research in Nursing*. London: RCN.

RCN (1976) *Code of Professional Conduct – a Discussion Document*. London: RCN.

RCN (1979) *Charter and Byelaws*. London: RCN.

Ramsey P (1965) *Deeds and Rules in Christian Ethics*. Cambridge: Cambridge University Press.

Ramsey P (1970) *The Patient as Person: Explorations in Medical Ethics*. New Haven, Connecticut: Yale University Press.

Ramsey P (1978) *Ethics at the Edges of Life: Medical and Legal Intersections*. New Haven, Connecticut: Yale University Press.

Reich WT (1978) *Encyclopedia of Bioethics*: 4 Volumes. London: Macmillan.

Reiser SJ, Dyck AJ and Curran WT (1977) *Ethics in Medicine*. Boston: MIT Press.

Riemen D (1986) The essential structure of a caring interaction: doing phenomenology. In: Munhall PL and Oiler CJ (eds) *Nursing Research: a Qualitative Perspective*. Norwalk, Connecticut: Appleton-Century-Crofts, 85–108.

Roach MS (1984) *Caring, the Human Mode of Being, Implications for Nursing*. Toronto: University of Toronto.

Roach Sr MS (1987) *The Human Act of Caring: a Blueprint for the Health Professions*. Ottawa, Ontario: Canadian Hospital Association.

Robb B (1967) *Sans Everything*. London: Nelson.

Rogers CR (1977) *On Personal Power*. London: Constable.

Rumbold G (1986) *Ethics in Nursing Practice*. London: Baillière Tindall.

Salvage J (1985) *The Politics of Nursing*. London: Heinemann.

Samarel N (1989) Caring for the living and the dying: a study of role transition. *International Journal of Nursing Studies* **26**(4) 313–326.

Sampson C (1982) *The Neglected Ethic: Religious and Cultural Factors in the Care of Patients*. London: McGraw-Hill.

Sarason SB (1985) *Caring and Compassion in Clinical Practice*. London: Jossey-Bass.

Sartre J-P (1973) *Existentialism and Humanism*. Translated P. Mairet. London: Methuen.

Schein E (1984) Coming to a new awareness of organisational culture. *Sloan Management Review* **25**(2) 3–16.

Schmidt JA and Wolfe JS (1980) The mentor partnership: Discovery of professionalism. *NASPA Journal* **17**: 45–51.

Schorck R (1980) A question of honesty in nursing practice. *Journal of Advanced Nursing* **5**(2) 135–148.

Schulman ED (1982) *Intervention in Human Services: A Guide to Skills and Knowledge*. 3rd edn. St Louis, Toronto: CV Mosby.

Scorer G and Wing A (eds) (1979) *Decision Making in Medicine: the Practice of its Ethics*. London: Arnold.

Scott R (1981) *The Body as Property*. London: Viking Press.

Scrivenger M (1987) Ethics, etiquette and the law. *Nursing Times* **83**(42) 28–29.

Sedgwick P (1982) *Psycho Politics*. London: Pluto Press.

Shropshire CO (1981) Group experiential learning in adult education. *Journal of Continuing Education in Nursing* **12**(6) 5–9.

Sieghart P (1985) Professions as the conscience of society. *Journal of Medical Ethics* **11**(3) 117–122.

Simmons D (1982) *Personal Valuing: an Introduction*. Chicago: Helson Hall.

Simon SB, Howe LW and Kirschenbaum H (1978) *Values Clarification: A Handbook of Practical Strategies for Teachers and Students*. New York: A and W Visual Library.

Stephenson M and Moran L (1987) The dilemma of ethics. *Senior Nurse* 793) 47–48.

Stitch TF (1983) Experiential therapy. *Journal of Experiential Education* **5**(3) 23–30.

Stockwell F (1972) *The Unpopular Patient*. London: RCN.

Styles MM (1982) *On Nursing: Towards a new endowment*. St Louis: CV Mosby.

Tate BL (1977) *The Nurse's Dilemma: Ethical Considerations in Nursing Practice*. Geneva; ICN Code.

Thiroux JP (1980) *Ethics, Theory and Practice*. 2nd edn. Encino, California: Glencoe Publishing.

Thompson IA, Melia K and Boyd K (1983) *Nursing Ethics*. Edinburgh: Churchill Livingstone.

Thomson WAR (1977) *A Dictionary of Medical Ethics and Practice*. Bristol: Wright.

Tillich P (1963) *Morality and Beyond*. London: Harper and Row.

Toulmin S (1958) *The Place of Reason in Ethics*. Cambridge: Cambridge University Press.

Townesend P and Davidson N (1982) *Inequalities in Health*. Harmondsworth: Penguin.

Tschudin V (1986) *Ethics in Nursing: the Caring Relationship*. London: Heinemann.

UKCC (1984) *Code of Professional Conduct*. London: UKCC.

Van Hooft S (1987) Caring and professional commitment. *Australian Journal of Advanced Nursing* **4**(4) 29–38.

Veatch RM (1977) *Case Studies in Medical Ethics*. Cambridge, Mass: Harvard University Press.

Vousden M (1987) Top secret code? *Nursing Times* **83**(42) 25–27.

Warnock M (1970) *Existentialism*. London: Oxford University Press.

Watson J (1979) *Nursing: The Philosophy and Science of Caring*. New York: Little, Brown and Co.

Watson J (1985) *Nursing: Human Science and Human Care: A Theory of Nursing*. Norwalk, Connecticut: Appleton-Century-Crofts.

White R (1985) *Political Issues in Nursing*. Chichester: Wiley.

Williams B (1976) *Morality: An Introduction to Ethics*. Cambridge: Cambridge University Press.

Wright D (1971) *The Psychology of Moral Behaviour*. Harmondsworth: Penguin.

Young AP (1981) *Legal Problems in Nursing Practice*. London: Harper and Row.

# Index